Muscle Diseases

This volume is a how-to guide on the clinical assessment and investigation of patients presenting with muscle-related symptoms. Featuring a case-based approach, this accessible text is suitable for a wide range of clinical specialists who see patients presenting with both common and rare muscle diseases.

Muscle diseases are often initially missed or misdiagnosed, as they are uncommon disorders and can present in a variety of ways, often mimicking other more common disorders. Careful assessment of the history, physical examination and appropriate choice of investigations is therefore essential to reaching a diagnosis and providing short- and long-term effective management plans. Key features of this resource include:

- A case-based approach using real cases seen in clinical practice and highlighting different clinical presentations
- Case vignettes that cover patient history, examination, investigations, diagnosis and discussion points to assist the reader in developing a mental framework for thinking about muscle disease and approaching diagnosis
- The relevant investigations (including muscle biopsy, neurophysiology and muscle imaging) required for each clinical scenario, aiding the clinician in clinicopathological correlation
- Being concise, practical and complemented by a wide range of figures to enhance understanding

Patients with muscle diseases may be referred to one of several medical or surgical specialties, including neurology, rheumatology, neuropathology, neurophysiology, cardiology, respiratory medicine, intensive care medicine, gastroenterology, ophthalmology, orthopaedic and spinal surgery, before the correct diagnosis is considered. This accessible text is an ideal resource for clinicians.

T0386573

Muscle Diseases

A Guide to Differential Diagnosis, Investigation and Management

Andria Merrison and Stefen Brady

Image Editor Kathryn Urankar

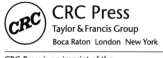

CRC Press
Taylor & Francis Group
Boca Raton London New York

CRC Press is an imprint of the
Taylor & Francis Group, an **informa** business

Designed cover image: Kathryn Urankar
First edition published 2025
by CRC Press
2385 NW Executive Center Drive, Suite 320, Boca Raton FL 33431

and by CRC Press
4 Park Square, Milton Park, Abingdon, Oxon, OX14 4RN
CRC Press is an imprint of Taylor & Francis Group, LLC

Library of Congress Cataloging-in-Publication Data

Names: Merrison, Andria, editor. | Brady, Stefen, editor.
Title: Muscle diseases : a guide to differential diagnosis, investigation and management / [edited by] Andria Merrison and Stefen Brady ; image editor, Kathryn Urankar.
Other titles: Muscle diseases (Merrison)
Description: First edition. | Boca Raton, FL : CRC Press, 2025. | Includes bibliographical references and index.
Identifiers: LCCN 2024017755 (print) | LCCN 2024017756 (ebook) | ISBN 9781138368330 (hardback) | ISBN 9781138368026 (paperback) | ISBN 9780429429323 (ebook)
Subjects: MESH: Neuromuscular Diseases--diagnosis | Neuromuscular Diseases--therapy | Diagnosis, Differential | Case Reports
Classification: LCC RC925.55 (print) | LCC RC925.55 (ebook) | NLM WE 550 | DDC 616.7/44--dc23/eng/20241112
LC record available at https://lccn.loc.gov/2024017755
LC ebook record available at https://lccn.loc.gov/2024017756

ISBN: 9781138368330 (hbk)
ISBN: 9781138368026 (pbk)
ISBN: 9780429429323 (ebk)

DOI: 10.1201/9780429429323

Typeset in Minion
by Deanta Global Publishing Services, Chennai, India

My thanks go to my inspirational parents, gorgeous husband, wonderful daughters (Alice, Grace & Olivia); as well to our patient publishers (Georgia & Miranda) and all the patients and families that we have served.

—Andria Merrison

There are many people to thank for putting up with and supporting me while I was writing this book and they know who they are. However, I have one specific dedication, come apology, to a friend and colleague. She suggested, many times, that we write a book like this when we were trainees together in London. However, back then I had neither the time nor probably the necessary experience and ultimately our paths diverged. Hopefully this dedication will make up for my reticence.

—Stefen Brady

CONTENTS

Contents

PREFACE

This book serves as a window into the world of diagnosis, treatment and care for people living with neuromuscular conditions. It introduces neuromuscular conditions and the diagnostic armamentarium available, as well as possible management approaches and treatment options.

Presented as a series of clinical cases – each set out in terms of history, examination and investigation findings – the reader is led through the clinical journey in each case. It can be approached as a number of tests – probing one's knowledge of the neuromuscular clinical arena (should the reader wish to take on this challenge) – before delving into the diagnosis and discussion that follows. Alternatively, it is a gentle walk through the key areas of neuromuscular clinical practice – each case providing a means of structuring and remembering clinical knowledge.

We have been privileged to have shared some of the experiences of many people living with neuromuscular conditions in very different ways. We hope to be able to share some of the passion, inspiration and understanding that we have been given in a way that is both accessible and useful to clinicians seeking to know more about this area of medicine and in turn help others living with these conditions.

ABOUT THE EDITORS

Andria Merrison, MA, MBChB, MD, FRCP
Andria Merrison is a Consultant Neurologist based in North Bristol NHS Trust and is the Director of the South West Neuromuscular Operational Delivery Network and the Bristol Motor Neurone Disease Centre. She trained at Gonville and Caius College, Cambridge University and the University of Bristol. In her role as a board member of the NHS England Neurosciences Clinical Reference Group, she led on a service specification for Neurology for NHS England. She is also an MRCP Part 2 Examination Board member, and Regional Advisor and Regional Specialty Advisor for the Royal College of Physicians.

Stefen Brady, BA, MB, BCh, BAO, MSc, DPhil, FRCP
Stefen Brady is a Consultant Neurologist and Clinical Lead of the Oxford Adult Muscle and Spinal Muscular Atrophy (SMA) Services, Department of Clinical Neurosciences, John Radcliffe Hospital, Oxford. He studied medicine at Trinity College Medical School, University of Dublin; and trained in neurology in Yorkshire. He completed a DPhil in clinical neurology at Keble College, University of Oxford. He is a committee member of the British Myology Society and has the honour of being Treasurer for the Oxford Muscle Symposium.

Image Editor:
Kathryn Urankar, BSc MBBS, FRCPA (Anat. Path; For Path); FRCPath (Neuropath)
Kathryn Urankar is a Consultant Neuropathologist based at North Bristol NHS Trust and is the muscle biopsy lead in the department of Neuropathology, both performing and interpreting muscle biopsies for the South-West region. She studied medicine at the University of Queensland in Brisbane, Australia and undertook her initial pathology training in Queensland with Pathology Queensland. She has subsequently worked in the fields of Forensic Pathology and Neuropathology in Australia, Canada and the United Kingdom as well as a brief stint at USCF learning from some of the best neuropathologists in the world. She currently holds the position of Chair of Examiners in Neuropathology for the Royal College of Pathologists of the United Kingdom and Head of School of Pathology for the Severn & Pennisula Deaneries.

LIST OF CONTRIBUTORS

Kezia Austin
North Bristol NHS Trust
Bristol, UK

Rajat Chowdhury
Oxford University Hospitals NHS
    Trust
Oxford, UK

Charlotte David
Barts Health NHS Trust
London, UK

Joel David
Oxford University Hospitals NHS
    Trust
Oxford, UK

Carl Fratter
Oxford University Hospitals NHS
    Trust
Oxford, UK

Harsha Gunawardena
North Bristol NHS Trust
Bristol, UK

Louisa Kent
Oxford University Hospitals NHS Trust
Oxford, UK

Maria Mirza
Royal Berkshire NHS Hospitals Trust
Berkshire, UK

Agyepong Oware
North Bristol NHS Trust
Bristol, UK

Sithara Ramdas
Oxford University Hospitals NHS
    Trust
Oxford, UK

Kate Sergeant
Oxford University Hospitals NHS
    Trust
Oxford, UK

Matthew Wells
North Bristol NHS Trust
Bristol, UK

Kathryn Urankar
North Bristol NHS Trust
Bristol, UK

INTRODUCTION

Muscle conditions form a fascinating area of medicine that lies in an ever-changing landscape. They encompass a wide range of diseases (over 60 named in the UK NHS specialised definition set) which present in a myriad of different ways. Over 50,000 people in the UK have one of this diverse group of genetic and acquired conditions that make up primary muscle disease and many more have muscle symptoms due to drugs or systemic disease. The important acquired muscle diseases include the inflammatory myopathies, which are treatable and so diagnosis must not be missed (or overdiagnosed and some other disorder treated inappropriately), as well as the drug-induced myopathies. Clinicians are often asked to assess patients with secondary muscle dysfunction due to ageing, immobility, critical illness or cancer.

Many neuromuscular conditions have a genetic basis, and advances in genetics has obviated the need for more invasive tests in many cases. There is an increasing ability to make a diagnosis by identifying causative genes; through linkage studies, whole genome or exome sequencing in cohorts of patients with specific features. However, there are likely to be many more genetic abnormalities that will in time be confirmed to be associated with disease (many more than the few we routinely analyse now), and there may be involvement of more than one gene or a variety of genetic mechanisms at play to cause disease. Patients may also present with very different phenotypes, even with the same genotype in the same family. Careful assessment of the history, physical examination and appropriate choice of investigations are therefore essential to reaching a diagnosis and providing short- and long-term effective management plans.

Muscle conditions impair mobility and frequently cause cardiorespiratory complications. The range of their age of onset is very wide; patients may die during early life, face lifelong disability or present with late-onset muscle weakness. Distinguishing myopathies from peripheral neuropathy, anterior horn cell dysfunction and neuromuscular junction disorders can be challenging.

Providing excellent care requires a multidisciplinary team dedicated to helping people living with neuromuscular conditions. Careful co-ordination of a variety of different medical and surgical specialisms is often essential for successful long-term management.

CLASSIFICATION OF MYOPATHIES IN ADULTS

Acquired		
Primary	Polymyositis	
	Dermatomyositis	
	Inclusion body myositis	
Secondary	Drugs and toxins	
	Connective tissue disease and other autoimmune disorders	
	Endocrine	
	Metabolic	
	Infections	
Inherited		
Muscular dystrophy	Myotonic dystrophy type 1 and 2	
	Dystrophinopathies: Duchenne and Becker muscular dystrophy	
	Facioscapulohumeral dystrophy	
	Limb girdle muscular dystrophies	
	Emery–Dreifuss muscular dystrophy	
	Oculopharyngeal muscular dystrophy	
Congenital myopathies	Nemaline	
	Core myopathies	
Myofibrillar myopathies		
Distal myopathies		
Metabolic myopathies	Glycogen metabolism: McArdle's	
	Fatty acid metabolism: CPT2 deficiency, acyl-CoA dehydrogenase deficiency	
Channelopathies	Non-dystrophic myotonias	
	Periodic paralysis	
Mitochondrial disease	Chronic progressive external ophthalmoplegia	

DIAGNOSTIC FEATURES OF MUSCLE CONDITIONS

Facial weakness	FSHD
	Myotonic dystrophy
	Inclusion body myositis
	Polymyositis
	Myasthenia gravis
Ophthalmoplegia/ptosis	Mitochondrial cytopathy (often without double vision)
	Thyroid myopathy
	Myasthenia gravis
Dysphagia	Inclusion body myositis
	Polymyositis
	Oculopharyngeal muscular dystrophy
	Motor neurone disease
	Myasthenia gravis/Lambert Eaton myasthenic syndrome, congenital myasthenia
Neck weakness	Myasthenia gravis
	Motor neurone disease
	Polymyositis
Myotonia	Myotonic dystrophy type 1 and 2
	Non-dystrophic myotonias (myotonia congenita, paramyotonia congenita)
Contractures	Emery–Dreifuss muscular dystrophy
	Limb girdle muscular dystrophy 2A (calpainopathy)
	Bethlem myopathy

ABBREVIATIONS

AD	autosomal dominant
ALT	alanine aminotransferase
AR	autosomal recessive
AST	aspartate aminotransferase
BiPAP	bilevel positive airway pressure
BMD	Becker muscular dystrophy
CK	creatine kinase
COX	cytochrome c oxidase
CPAP	continuous positive airway pressure
DM	myotonic dystrophy
DMD	Duchenne muscular dystrophy
ECG	electrocardiogram
EDMD	Emery–Dreifuss muscular dystrophy
EM	electron microscopy
EMG	electromyography
FKRP	fukutin-related protein
FSHD	facioscapulohumeral muscular dystrophy
GSD	glycogen storage disorder
IBM	inclusion body myositis
IHC	immunohistochemical
IIM	idiopathic inflammatory myopathy
IMNM	immune-mediated necrotising myopathy
LGMD	limb girdle muscular dystrophy
MAC	membrane attack complex
MELAS	mitochondrial encephalomyopathy, lactic acidosis and stroke-like episodes
MHC	major histocompatibility complex
MLPA	multiplex ligation-dependent probe amplification
MRC	Medical Research Council
MRI	magnetic resonance imaging
NADH	nicotinamide adenine dinucleotide
NCS	nerve conduction study
NGS	next-generation sequencing
PAS	periodic acid-Schiff
SDH	succinate dehydrogenase
SMA	spinal muscular atrophy
SR	sarcoplasmic reticulum
STIR	short-tau inversion recovery
TAM	tubular aggregate myopathy
TAs	tubular aggregates

CHAPTER 1

HISTORY

Andria Merrison

Clinicians encounter people living with muscle conditions presenting in isolation or as part of a multisystem disorder. More than 50,000 people in the UK have one of a diverse group of genetic and acquired conditions that make up the primary muscle disorders. These include muscular dystrophies, and congenital, metabolic, mitochondrial and inflammatory myopathies. An even greater number of people are affected by secondary muscle problems due to drugs, ageing, immobility, critical illness, systemic metabolic disorders and cancer.

Over 85% of neuromuscular conditions, including genetic muscle problems, present in adult life. Advances in genetics have led to greatly improved diagnostics and new therapies for muscle conditions (including dystrophinopathies, spinal muscular atrophy and others). Respiratory and cardiac complications of muscle disorders are common and early recognition and effective management can save lives, reduce morbidity and improve quality of life.

Distinguishing myopathies from peripheral neuropathies (hereditary or inflammatory neuropathy), anterior horn cell diseases (amyotrophic lateral sclerosis, spinal muscular atrophy or Kennedy's disease) and neuromuscular junction disorders (myasthenic syndromes) requires careful clinical evaluation. This includes diligent history taking, thorough examination and implementation of appropriate investigations.

DOI: 10.1201/9780429429323-1

HISTORY

A number of diagnostic clues may be derived from the history on the basis of the age of onset, family history, rate of progression/temporal pattern of weakness and pattern of muscle involvement. The following may be reported by the patient (or subsequently become evident): weakness, myalgia, wasting, hypertrophy, muscle stiffness, cramps, myoglobinuria and/or respiratory or cardiac involvement.

Age of onset

- Duchenne muscular dystrophy presents at <5 years, inclusion body myositis generally in midlife and mitochondrial disease at any age.
- Dermatomyositis is much more common than polymyositis in childhood.
- Many muscular dystrophies, such as facioscapulohumeral, myotonic and limb girdle muscular dystrophy tend to present in adolescence or early adult life, but both late and young onset are recognised.
- Childhood features: Reduced fetal movements in pregnancy, "floppy baby", feeding or breathing problems, delayed motor milestones and limited sporting achievements can all point to a congenital or childhood-onset disorder. These features alone may not distinguish a muscle problem from a neuromuscular junction or peripheral nerve disorder.

Family history

- The family history may reveal an autosomal recessive/dominant, X-linked or mitochondrial pattern of inheritance.
- Some conditions show genetic anticipation (e.g., myotonic dystrophy), manifesting with increasing severity in subsequent generations.
- Systemic features in other family members (e.g., early cataracts in myotonic dystrophy) may be the only manifestation of a condition in preceding generations.

Pattern of muscle involvement

The distribution of muscle weakness can be an important clue to the diagnosis.

- Facial involvement: Consider facioscapulohumeral muscular dystrophy, oculopharyngeal muscular dystrophy and sometimes inflammatory myositis or mitochondrial myopathy.
- Ophthalmoplegia: Check for fatiguability to exclude myasthenia gravis. If there is no fatiguability the common causes are mitochondrial disease (often without double vision despite significant dysconjugate gaze), oculopharyngeal muscular dystrophy and myotubular myopathy. Ptosis may be associated with ophthalmoplegia and be evident in isolation in these conditions and congenital myopathies.
- Proximal (limb girdle) muscle weakness is the commonest presentation and has many causes: muscular dystrophy, metabolic or mitochondrial myopathy, polymyositis and dermatomyositis.

- Inclusion body myositis usually affects the quadriceps muscles (causing proximal lower limb weakness) and the long finger and wrist flexors (causing distal weakness in the upper limbs).
- Isolated distal weakness is usually neurogenic in origin (peripheral neuropathy, anterior horn cell disease, radiculopathy) but can occur in myotonic dystrophy, myofibrillar myopathy and some other congenital myopathies.
- Bulbar weakness (dysphagia/dysarthria): Consider myotonic dystrophy, inclusion body myositis, inflammatory, mitochondrial and endocrine myopathies, and oculopharyngeal muscular dystrophy.

Weakness

Weakness will lead to a range of functional difficulties, which may be progressive. Progression is usually gradual and linear, but the experience of losing the ability to do something that one could previously do is often stepwise. This may include difficulty with activities above shoulder height (reaching into overhead cupboards or brushing/washing hair) or problems with grip strength (opening jars, doing up buttons or using a screwdriver). Negotiating stairs, rising from a seated/squat or supine position, standing on tiptoes or on heels can all be difficult, and foot drop and falls can occur.

Facial weakness is usually bilateral and symmetrical and can often go unnoticed or unreported. It can lead to difficulty whistling, blowing up balloons, using a straw or dysarthria. Difficulty with eye closure during sleep may indicate more severe facial weakness and protection of the cornea (with eye gels/lubricants) is essential to preserving vision.

Myalgia

Myalgia is a common complaint and often not due to muscle disease but instead due to other systemic problems, including infection, arthritis and polymyalgia rheumatica. Myalgia without weakness, myoglobinuria or a rise in plasma creatine kinase and normal electromyography is unlikely to be due to muscle disease. Muscle conditions where myalgia is commonly a feature include inflammatory myopathies, myotonic dystrophy (and non-dystrophic myotonia), hypothyroidism, vitamin D deficiency and drug-induced myopathy. Myalgia precipitated by exercise occurs in metabolic and mitochondrial myopathies, dystrophinopathies, myotonic dystrophy (particularly type 2) and sometimes in inflammatory myopathies.

Muscle stiffness

Although some degree of muscle stiffness is common in muscle disorders, very marked stiffness and difficulty with muscle relaxation may be caused by myotonia. Some drugs, e.g., beta blockers, can exacerbate myotonia. In myotonia congenita, there is a worsening with rest and reduced myotonia with exercise, known as the "warm-up phenomenon". In paramyotonia congenita, there is exacerbation with exercise and with cold, known as "paradoxical myotonia".

Cramps

Cramps are more commonly seen in neurogenic disorders. If they are very prominent, one should consider drug-induced myopathy, metabolic muscle disease, mitochondrial myopathy or hypothyroidism.

Myoglobinuria

Myoglobin released from damaged muscle can colour the urine dark brown/black. This can occur in glycogenoses, fatty acid disorders, mitochondrial respiratory chain dysfunction, malignant hyperthermia, dystrophinopathies, inflammatory myopathy, infection, ischaemia, trauma, alcohol and drug-induced myopathy.

Respiratory and cardiac muscle involvement

Respiratory and cardiac muscle may be affected to differing degrees and at different stages in a variety of neuromuscular conditions. This can lead to reduced exercise tolerance, which may be difficult to establish in patients who are already immobile.

- Respiratory symptoms arise due to diaphragmatic, intercostal muscle and upper airway weakness (and in a minority of cases centrally driven problems, e.g., some people living with myotonic dystrophy). The hypercapnia that results leads to many of these symptoms. They include dyspnoea, orthopnoea, early morning headache and excessive daytime somnolence.
- Cardiac symptoms are due to dysrhythmia and/or cardiac failure: syncope, palpitations, dyspnoea and peripheral neuropathy.

General anaesthesia

Some myopathies are associated with malignant hyperthermia (e.g., central core or RyR1-associated myopathy) or similar reactions (e.g., periodic paralysis). Anaesthesia may also unmask previously unrecognised cardiorespiratory insufficiency.

CHAPTER 2

MUSCLE EXAMINATION

Stefen Brady

Taking an accurate history and performing a detailed physical examination are the most helpful "tests" a clinician has in the diagnosis of myopathies. With experience, pattern recognition resulting from detailed history, observational skills and thorough physical examination often enables one to confidently make a clinical diagnosis, which guides the selection of appropriate supportive tests and genetic analysis. The physical examination of a patient with a suspected myopathy differs slightly from the standard neurological examination. As usual, it involves a combination of inspection, functional assessment, tone, manual muscle testing, sensory examination, coordination and reflex testing. In addition, it is worth spending a bit of time examining the skin (see later), joints for hyperlaxity and contractures, and cardiorespiratory systems.

DOI: 10.1201/9780429429323-2

INSPECTION

Inspection begins with observing the patient sitting in the waiting room for characteristic facial features associated with myopathies such as myotonic dystrophy type 1 (DM1; ptosis, frontal balding, and wasting of masseter and temporalis) and facioscapulohumeral muscular dystrophy (FSHD; Bell's phenomenon and lower facial atrophy with prominence of the lips and cheeks). The presence of pelvic girdle weakness is suggested by the patient using their hands and arms to help them rise. Those with very severe pelvic girdle weakness may perform a modified Gower manoeuvre, which can look very dramatic to the unknowing observer. Here the patient places their hands on the floor in front of their chair and lifts themselves from the chair by weighting their arms whilst locking their legs straight. Once in this position (a forward fold), they rotate to face the chair which they then use, in addition to their legs, to climb up to achieve a standing position.

Next, take note of the patient's posture and gait. Those with marked ptosis will tip their head back to see under lowered eyelids. The normal position of the hand when walking is with the thumb pointing in the direction of travel. However, those with periscapular muscle weakness, e.g., FSHD, walk with the dorsum of the hand pointing in the direction of travel and the thumb pointing in towards the thigh of the same side.

A variety of different gaits may be observed in neurology clinics. It is slightly simpler in the adult muscle clinic with four main patterns of gait to be aware of:

    i. Waddling and hyperlordotic gait because of pelvic girdle weakness
    ii. Toe-walking due to the presence of ankle contractures
    iii. Steppage due to weakness of ankle dorsiflexion
    iv. Stiff-legged due to hyperextension (retroflexion) of the knee to compensate for weakness of knee extension

These patterns are not mutually exclusive and more than one can be observed in a single patient.

Myopathies can produce many signs in the head and neck (Table 2.1), particularly involving the extraocular and periocular muscles. Those to take note of include miosis (tubular aggregate myopathy [TAM]), ptosis (DM1, oculopharyngeal muscular dystrophy [OPMD], congenital myopathies, and mitochondrial myopathy), ophthalmoparesis without diplopia (OPMD, mitochondrial myopathy, and congenital myopathies), and cataracts (DM1 and 2, mitochondrial disease, and myofibrillar myopathy). Periocular weakness may be suggested by Bell's phenomenon. Muscle atrophy is seen in DM1 (temporalis, masseter, and sternocleidomastoid) and FSHD (perioral muscle atrophy resulting in prominence of the lips and cheeks). Orobulbar signs are an uncommon feature of adult myopathies, but dysphonia can accompany congenital myopathy and dysarthria in DM1. Perioral fasciculation suggests spinobulbar muscular atrophy (SBMA; Kennedy's disease), tongue atrophy and fasciculation spinal muscular atrophy (SMA) and SBMA (after ruling out the motor neurone disease), and tongue

Table 2.1 Clinical signs of myopathy in the head and neck

Signs in the head and neck	Possible diagnoses
Miosis	Tubular aggregate myopathy (TAM)
Cataracts	Myotonic dystrophies type 1 and 2 (DM1 and 2) Myofibrillar myopathy
Pigmentary retinopathy	Mitochondrial disease
Optic atrophy	Mitochondrial disease
Ophthalmoparesis	Congenital myopathy (CM) Mitochondrial disease Oculopharyngeal muscular dystrophy (OPMD)
Ptosis	Mitochondrial disease DM1 and 2 CM OPMD
Facial weakness	CM Congenital DM1 Facioscapulohumeral muscular dystrophy (FSHD)
Temporalis, masseter and sternocleidomastoid wasting	DM1
Tongue atrophy and fasciculation	Spinal muscular atrophy (SMA) Spinobulbar muscular atrophy (SBMA; Kennedy's disease)
Tongue hypertrophy	Duchenne and Becker muscular dystrophy Pompe disease Limb girdle muscular dystrophy type 9 (LGMD R9, *FKRP*)

hypertrophy is observed in muscular dystrophy and the glycogen storage disorder Pompe disease.

With the patient undressed, there is a further opportunity to observe their gait, inspect for fasciculation, and to look for generalised or focal muscle atrophy or hypertrophy. Pectoral muscle wasting in FSHD is evidenced by the presence of a horizontal axillary crease, while atrophy of the volar forearms is commonly seen in inclusion body myositis (IBM). Calf hypertrophy is most commonly associated with Duchenne and Becker muscular dystrophies (DMD and BMD) but can be present in several other hereditary myopathies. Generalised muscle hypertrophy may be observed in myotonia congenita, *RYR1*-related myopathy and very rarely DM1. Skeletal changes (kyphoscoliosis, increased lumbar lordosis) and dermatological signs are useful in directing the clinician to particular diagnoses. Minor degrees of scoliosis and spinal rigidity are demonstrated by asking the patient to touch their toes while standing. Prior to examining the patient on the couch, the examiner should inspect the patient's back for scapular winging (aka scapula alata).

Manual muscle assessment

Searching for muscle weakness is best done in a systematic head-to-toe fashion. How best to record the severity of weakness is down to the individual. Each system has its pros and cons. Over time, I have become more enamoured with a simple system that I acquired from a mentor: mild weakness (Medical Research Council [MRC] –5 to 4/5), moderate weakness (MRC 3/5), and severe weakness (MRC <3/5). Mild bilateral facial weakness can be very difficult to identify unless specifically sought. Subtle periocular weakness may only be identified by a patient's inability to fully bury their eyelashes, while perioral muscle atrophy and weakness may be evidenced by detection of a transverse smile and/or prominent lips and cheeks. The same can be said for mild degrees of bilateral ptosis. A clue to its presence is frontalis overactivity.

Several patterns of weakness of are often described in myopathies:

i. Duchenne and Becker type: neck flexion weakness accompanied by hip girdle weakness greater than shoulder girdle sometimes accompanied by weakness of ankle dorsiflexion.

ii. Limb girdle weakness: hip girdle weakness greater than shoulder girdle.

iii. FSHD type (aka scapuloperoneal): periocular and perioral weakness with scapular winging and weakness of ankle dorsiflexion.

iv. Distal weakness: predominant involvement of the extensor or flexor muscle groups of the distal upper limb (e.g., Welander myopathy or myasthenic syndromes) or, more commonly, the distal lower limb (most commonly weakness of ankle dorsiflexion, which is found in many hereditary myopathies, and much less frequently weakness of ankle plantarflexion, which is observed in dysferlinopathy).

v. OPMD type: (ptosis with or without ophthalmoparesis), dysphagia, and proximal weakness.

vi. Emery–Dreifuss muscular dystrophy (EDMD): scapuloperoneal weakness with prominent joint contractures.

vii. Distal and proximal weakness: observed in inclusion body myositis where early weakness of finger flexion is identified in conjunction with weakness of knee extension.

viii. Generalised asthenia: slim muscles associated with a mild generalised weakness, as observed in congenital myopathy.

Mild asymmetry of strength is not unusual, but marked asymmetry is suggestive of FSHD and IBM. Clinically, it can be difficult to differentiate a length-dependent motor neuropathy and a distal myopathy. A useful sign of the underlying pathology is the presence or absence of extensor digitorum brevis on the dorsum of the foot, which is typically atrophied in neuropathy but preserved in distal myopathy.

It is easy to overlook the abdomen, but don't! There are clues to the diagnosis to be found here too. Abdominal muscle weakness may result in asymptomatic asymmetric bulges of the abdominal wall when seated or standing. Beevor sign describes the cranial movement of the umbilicus when the recumbent patient lifts their head from the examination couch. Movement of the umbilicus is due to weakness of the lower abdominal muscles. It was originally described in patients with thoracic spinal cord injury. However, it is often observed in FSHD. Although neither 100 per cent sensitive nor specific, its presence is highly supportive of this diagnosis. Sometimes the umbilicus moves caudally, indicative of upper abdominal muscle weakness.

Sensation and coordination

Impaired coordination is a commonly reported symptom in individuals with a myopathy. For the most part, it is usually the result of muscle weakness rather than attesting to the presence of a concomitant neuropathy or cerebellar involvement. For most patients, a detailed sensory examination is unnecessary. A usually more than adequate screen is to test the vibration and joint position senses. If these are abnormal, further more detailed examination may be required. Sensory signs are found in mitochondrial disease, myofibrillar myopathy and very rarely in disorders of fatty acid oxidation (i.e., metabolic myopathy). There are many more detailed texts on performing an examination for cerebellar disease. I will limit myself to saying that cerebellar signs in combination with weakness are highly suggestive of mitochondrial disease.

Reflexes

Tendon reflexes may be normal, reduced or absent in myopathies. With mild myopathic weakness, tendon reflexes should be present. As the severity of weakness increases, tendon reflexes can reduce and may sometimes disappear altogether. Upper motor neuron (UMN) signs are never observed in a myopathy (bar hyperreflexia in hyperthyroidism and mitochondrial disease with central nervous system involvement). If present, UMN signs are indicative of an alternative diagnosis, such as motor neurone disease, or much less likely (if no reason is evident on history such as previous stroke) a second diagnosis.

Myotonia plus

Excluding cramps, which are a neurogenic phenomenon, there are three abnormal muscle contractions to be aware of: myotonia and paramyotonia, myoedema, and rippling muscle. Myotonia, delayed muscle relaxation, is the most frequently encountered. It is observed by asking the patient to forcibly close their eyes or make a fist before opening it quickly. The affected patient will struggle to open their eyes or fist quickly on initial command. However, with repeated action, the myotonia lessens and performing the requested movement becomes easier. With paramyotonia, the movement does not get easier and can worsen with repetition. Myotonia can be elicited by striking the origin of the finger extensors in the forearm or thenar eminence with a tendon hammer. Although clinical myotonia (myotonia on examination rather than with electromyography [EMG]) can be demonstrated in a few different myopathies, because of its prevalence, DM1 should be the presumed diagnosis whilst awaiting genetic confirmation. Myoedema is indicative of hypothyroidism. It is the production of a lump in the muscle (mounding of muscle) when a muscle is struck with a tendon hammer. The lump resolves over a few seconds. Rippling muscle is a wave of contraction spreading across a muscle in response to percussion or stretching. It is observed with pathogenic variants in *CAV3* and can be autoimmune in origin. Both myo-edema and rippling muscle are electrically silent on EMG.

Dermatological features of muscle disease

Skin diseases are relatively frequent in muscle diseases and are often highly specific to particular diagnoses. The most well-known are those associated with idiopathic inflammatory myopathies (IIMs). Findings in dermatomyositis include but aren't limited to periocular heliotrope rash and oedema, erythematous photosensitive rashes over the anterior chest (V-sign), shoulders and upper back (shawl sign), and lateral thigh (holster sign), Gottron's papules and sign, ragged hypertrophied cuticles, dilated nailfold capillaries, and subcutaneous limb oedema. Patients with antisynthetase syndrome may report and demonstrate Raynaud's phenomenon and mechanic's hands (fissuring of the skin, particularly the ulnar edge of the little finger). Sclerodactyly may be seen in overlap myositis. Lesser-known cutaneous changes associated with myopathies include (i) radiation changes associated with radiotherapy-induced myopathy; (ii) hypertrophic and keloid scarring, and hyperkeratosis pilaris with collagen VI-related myopathies; (iii) ichthyosis in neutral lipid storage disease (aka Chanarin–Dorfman syndrome); (iv) epidermolysis bullosa in *PLEC*-related muscle disease; (v) pilomatrixomata in DM1; (vi) lipomatosis in mitochondrial disease associated with the pathogenic point variant m.8344A>G; and (vii) lipoatrophy in *LMNA*-related myopathy.

Final comment

The physical examination of a patient with a presumed myopathy can seem daunting, but it becomes easier and quicker with practice. If one piece of advice can be offered, it is to always examine the patient's back for scapular winging, an incredibly helpful and often missed diagnostic sign.

CHAPTER 3

SEROLOGICAL TESTS

Stefen Brady

Creatine kinase (CK; aka creatine phosphokinase) is the most widely serological test employed in the investigation of a myopathy. It is vital in the transformation of adenosine diphosphate (ADP) to adenosine triphosphate (ATP), the energy currency of cells. There are several isoforms of CK: CK-MM, CK-MB, CK-BB and CK-MiMi. The predominant isoform in serum is the skeletal muscle form, CK-MM. CK-MiMi, the mitochondrial isoform, is not normally present in serum. The routine measurement of CK does not distinguish between different CK isoforms. Infrequently, it is necessary to determine the subtype of CK contributing to hyperCKaemia. To do this, CK electrophoresis is required.

Although measurement of the serum CK is an easily performed and helpful investigation, it has limitations. Although the largest pool of CK in the body is skeletal muscle, there are non-myopathic, sometimes physiological causes for a raised CK, including a patient's race, sex, and age, or pathological, such as impaired clearance of CK in chronic renal disease, trauma, and neuropathy or following an acute myocardial infarction. The CK level is normal in many primary myopathies and the level of CK elevation is not indicative of disease severity. Monitoring CK levels has limited use except in the management of rhabdomyolysis and monitoring response to treatment of idiopathic inflammatory myopathies (IIMs). A rising CK indicates an impending relapse of a previously treated IIM and, usefully, this normally precedes clinical symptoms or signs.

A number of other serological markers are elevated in myopathies, including alanine and aspartate transaminase (ALT and AST), lactate dehydrogenase (LDH), aldolase and troponin. There is no reason to prefer any of these over CK. It is important to remember that ALT and AST are present in skeletal muscle and thus their elevation is not always indicative of liver disease. Troponins T and I are commonly measured with presumed cardiac disease. However, troponin T is not cardiac-specific and can also be elevated in myopathies.

Excluding testing for serum antibodies, there are a few other serological tests that have been used in the diagnosis of myopathies. These are mentioned here for completeness, though many have been or are being relegated to historical texts because of widespread access to whole-exome and/or whole-genome sequencing. Such tests include the non-ischaemic forearm exercise test for McArdle disease, white cell alpha-glucosidase in Pompe disease, carnitine and acylcarnitine profiles, plasma amino acids and urinary organic acids for metabolic myopathies, Jordans' phenomenon (the presence of lipid-containing vacuoles in leucocytes)

DOI: 10.1201/9780429429323-3

in neutral lipid storage disorders, and the detection of acanthocytes in McLeod's disease. However, these tests retain real-world utility in helping to clarify the pathogenicity of variants of uncertain significance, which are often identified through genomic testing.

Finally, in the investigation of mitochondrial disease, the following serological tests may sometimes be requested: serum and cerebrospinal fluid (CSF) lactate, serum fibroblast growth factor 21 (FGF21) and growth differentiation factor 15 (GDF15). Although elevated levels of such markers are suggestive of a primary mitochondrial disease, none individually, or in conjunction, are highly sensitive or specific for the diagnosis. Instead, mitochondrial genetic testing and respiratory chain enzyme analysis are the preferred means for diagnosis.

CHAPTER 4

MUSCLE ANTIBODIES

Maria Mirza and Joel David

INTRODUCTION

The diagnosis of inflammatory myopathy is usually made based on clinical symptoms combined with detection of raised creatine kinase (CK) levels, elevated acute phase proteins like C-reactive protein and an increased erythrocyte sedimentation rate on serological testing. Antinuclear antibodies (ANAs) may or may not be positive. Electromyography, characteristic findings on muscle biopsy, and the detection of autoantibodies may further help support the diagnosis of an inflammatory myositis.

Autoantibodies play a fundamental role in the diagnosis and classification of idiopathic inflammatory myopathy (IIM). Around 80% of patients with IIM will have a relevant muscle-associated autoantibody. The autoantibodies summarised in Table 4.1 target both nuclear and cytoplasmic components of the muscle fibre leading to muscle damage. There are two main categories of autoantibodies: myositis-specific antibodies (MSAs) and myositis-associated antibodies

Table 4.1 Myositis antibodies and the associated clinical conditions

Myositis-specific antibodies (MSAs)	Antibody-associated condition
Anti-ARS; anti-Jo-1, anti-PL7, anti-PL12, anti-EJ, anti-OJ, anti-Ha, anti-Ks and anti-Zo	Antisynthetase syndrome
Anti-SRP and anti-HMGCR antibodies	Immune-mediated necrotising myopathy
Anti-Mi2, anti-TIF1 and anti-NXP2	DM
Anti-MDA5 and anti-SAE	Clinically amyopathic DM
Myositis-associated antibodies (MAAs)	**Antibody-associated condition**
Anti-Ro/SSA	PM overlap with Sjogren's syndrome, systemic sclerosis; overlap with anti-synthetase syndrome
Anti-PmScl	PM and SSc
Anti-Ku	PM and SSc
Anti-U1RNP	PM and SLE

Abbreviations: Anti-ARS, antisynthetase syndrome; PM, polymyositis; DM, dermatomyositis; SSc, systemic sclerosis; SLE, systemic lupus erythematosus.

DOI: 10.1201/9780429429323-4

(MAAs). MSAs are highly specific for IIM with a 90% specificity compared to MAAs, which only occur in 50% of affected patients. MAAs are often found in overlap syndromes which occur when a medical condition shares features of two rheumatological disorders, for example, polymyositis and systemic sclerosis (PM/SSc). There is limited documentation on the utility of autoantibodies in the classification criteria of IIM. This could be due to a scarcity of data prior to the introduction of such criteria. Autoantibodies serve as biomarkers of disease, and as diagnostic testing increases in capacity and efficiency, they will play a more integral role in the classification criteria of IIM (1).

Myositis-specific antibodies
Anti-aminoacyl tRNA synthetase (anti-ARS) antibodies

After inclusion body myositis (IBM), antisynthetase syndrome (ASS) is the most common IIM in adults. It is typified by the presence of anti-ARS antibodies. ARS are cytoplasmic enzymes that catalyse the binding of tRNA to amino acids during protein synthesis. Anti-Jo1 is present in 11% of patients with IIM with the remaining anti-ARS antibodies like anti-PL7, anti-PL12, anti-EJ, anti-OJ, anti-Ha, anti-Ks and anti-Zo found in only 3.5% of patients (2). Anti-Jo1 is found in 20–30% of patients with polymyositis (PM) and 60–70% of myositis associated with interstitial lung disease (ILD). In 2010, Connors et al. introduced formal criteria for ASS, proposing that there must be evidence for tRNA synthetase autoantibody in addition to one or more of the following clinical features: mechanic's hands, Raynaud's phenomenon, myositis, ILD, arthritis and/or unexplained fever (3).

Anti-SRP and anti-HMGCR antibodies

Immune-mediated necrotising myopathy (IMNM) is characterised by the presence of antibodies to signal recognition particle (anti-SRP) or to 3-hydroxy-3-methylglutaryl CoA reductase (anti-HMGCR). Histopathology often reveals marked muscle fibre necrosis with minimal inflammatory infiltrate. CK levels can be markedly elevated (maybe in excess of 10,000 IU/L). Clinically, there is profound proximal weakness with a slow response to conventional therapy (4).

SRP is a cytoplasmic ribonucleoprotein made of six polypeptides complexed with a single 7sl RNA, and involved in secretory protein recognition and DNA translocation across the rough endoplasmic reticulum. Anti-SRP antibodies are found in around 4% of polymyositis (PM) patients. These cases typically demonstrate rapidly progressive muscle weakness.

Anti-HMGCR antibodies occur in 3–8% of adults with IIM. 3-hydroxy-3-methylglutaryl-coenzyme A is a key part of cholesterol biosynthesis, which is inhibited by statin therapy. There is a previous history of statin exposure in 40–92% of patients with detectable levels of anti-HMGCR autoantibodies. Most cases show a female-predominance, adult-onset disease typified by subacute progressive proximal weakness. Fatigue and myalgia are reported in 20–60% of patients. Anti-HMGCR myopathy classically affects the skeletal muscle, and non-specific symptoms such as rash, arthritis and Raynaud's phenomenon are uncommon (5,6).

Anti-Mi2, anti-TIF-1 and anti-NXP2 antibodies
Anti-Mi2 antibody

Dermatomyositis (DM) is an idiopathic autoimmune inflammatory disorder typified by a weakness, elevated CK and characteristic cutaneous manifestations. The skin features are often a defining feature, and hallmarks of the disease include periorbital dusky violaceous erythema, violaceous erythema over the face (malar/butterfly facial rash), chest (V sign), or shoulders and back (shawl sign). Gottron's papules, i.e., red scaly bumps over the knuckles, elbows or knees, are a further diagnostic cutaneous manifestation of DM. In some cases, patients present with cutaneous disease with subclinical or even absent muscle disease (7).

Anti-Mi2 autoantibodies can be detected in 11–59% of cases of adult DM and 4–10% of cases of juvenile dermatomyositis (JDM). Anti-Mi2-related DM shows a favourable prognosis with mild muscle involvement, low associations with ILD and cancer, and a good response to immunosuppressive therapy. Anti-Mi2 targets nucleosome remodelling and deacetylase. The Rituximab in Myositis (RIM) trial was the first prospective, double-blind randomised trial in myositis and the largest clinical trial performed in the setting of inflammatory myositis. Rituximab was found to provide a significant steroid-sparing effect between the start and conclusion of the trial. Furthermore, the presence of anti-Mi2 was linked to a shorter time to improvement in response to rituximab (8).

Anti-TIF1-gamma antibody

Anti-TIF1-gamma autoantibodies were discovered by Targoff et al., who, in 2006, identified an antibody targeting a 155 KDa nuclear protein later identified as transcription intermediary factor 1-gamma (9). TIF1 is a tripartite motif-containing protein essential in cellular pathways central to cell proliferation, apoptosis, and the innate immune system. Cutaneous involvement is a key finding in 13% of cases of adult DM and in 22–29% of cases of JDM which show positivity for anti-TIF1-gamma antibodies. A link between anti-TIF1 antibody-positive DM and cancer was identified in a meta-analysis undertaken by Trallero-Araguas et al. in 2006. This study revealed 78% sensitivity and 89% specificity in the diagnosis of an underlying myositis-associated cancer (10). Patients with anti-TIF1-gamma antibody-positive DM are less frequently afflicted by Raynaud's phenomenon, arthritis, calcinosis and ILD. However, pruritus, severe cutaneous disease and lower CK levels are more commonly seen in this group of myositis patients (11).

Anti-NXP2 antibody

Originally termed anti-MJ, anti-NXP2 antibodies target a 140-KDa nuclear protein called nuclear matrix protein 2 which plays a key role in P53-induced apoptosis following oncogenic stimulus. Anti-NXP2 antibodies occur in about 15% of patients with JDM. In anti-NXP2 antibody-positive JDM, severe cutaneous lesions are often observed along with calcinosis and muscle contractures. In adult men with DM, this antibody is associated with cancer (1).

Anti-MDA5 and anti-SAE antibodies

Anti-MDA5 antibodies were first described in a cohort of East Asian patients with clinically amyopathic myositis (81%) and rapidly progressive ILD (74%). These antibodies target IFN-induced melanoma differentiation-associated protein 5 (MDA5). In patients with this antibody, CK levels tend to be low and the disease is associated with a poor prognosis due to its association with respiratory failure. In addition, Sato et al. (2013) noted a link between anti-MDA5 antibodies and cutaneous ulceration in the nail folds and over the joint extensor surfaces (12).

Anti-SAE targets the small ubiquitin-like modifier-activating enzyme identified by Betteridge et al. (11). This autoantibody was observed in 6–8% of Caucasian patients with DM and even less frequently in Asian patients (2%). It is associated with HLA-DQB1*03 haplotype, which may explain the reduced frequency of the autoantibody among non-Caucasian patients. Dysphagia is seen in 78% of anti-SAE positive patients compared with 43% in anti-SAE negative group (11).

Myositis-associated autoantibodies (MAAs)

Anti-Ro/SSA

Anti-Ro autoantibodies are typically identified when PM or DM is associated with another connective tissue disease, for example, systemic sclerosis (SS). Anti-Ro/SSA antibody against the Ro52 subunit is the most conspicuous MAA, occurring in more than 30% of patients with IIM. Frequently, its presence over-laps with the presence of anti-ARS antibodies. The combination of anti-Ro/SSA antibodies with anti-Jo1 antibodies in ASS is associated with an increased risk of severe ILD, myositis, joint involvement and cancer. Myositis is reported to occur in 1–14% of primary Sjogren's syndrome cases. Anti-Ro and or anti-La antibodies occur frequently in PM/Sjogren's overlap syndrome, which comprises 5.3% of patients with PM (1).

Anti-PmScl

Anti-PmScl antibodies are one of the most common MAAs and are most commonly associated with PM and SS overlap. The presence of these autoantibodies suggests an increased risk of the development of ILD, inflammatory joint disease, mechanic's hands and Raynaud's phenomenon.

Anti-Ku

Anti-Ku antibodies are a relatively recently recognised autoantibody involved in IIM, particularly in cases previously thought to be autoantibody negative. Their presence is indicative of PM and SSc, having been reported in 28% of anti-Ku-positive patients. These patients tend to have a mild, glucocorticoid-responsive myopathy (11).

Anti-U1RNP

Anti-U1RNP antibodies are common in PM and SLE overlap syndrome and are also associated with anti-Jo1 antibodies in overlap myositis. Apart from myositis, these patients tend to have erosive arthritis, alopecia, ILD, oral ulcers and rarely glomerulonephritis (1).

Conclusion

Autoantibodies identified in cases of myositis are an expanding heterogeneous group. Detection of these autoantibodies is of great clinical utility, both diagnostic and prognostic, through the identification of those patients at increased risk of cancer and ILD. It is likely that the identification of specific autoantibodies in myositis will feature prominently in future classification or diagnostic criteria of IIM.

Further reading

1. Ghirardello A, Borella E, Beggio M, et al. Myositis autoantibodies and clinical phenotypes. *Auto Immun Highlights*. 2014;5(3):69–75.
2. McHugh N, Tansley S. Autoantibodies in myositis. *Nat Rev Rheumatol*. 2018;14:290–302.
3. Connors GR, Cristopher-Stine L, Oddis CV, et al. Interstitial lung disease associated with idiopathic inflammatory myopathies: What progress has been made in the past 35 years? *Chest*. 2010;138:1464–1474.
4. Lundberg IE, De Visser M, Werth VP. Classification of myositis. *Nat Rev Rheumatol*. 2018;14(5):269–278.
5. Mohassel P, Mammen AL. Anti-HMGCR Myopathy. *J Neuromuscular Dis*. 2018;5(1):11–20.
6. Selva-O'Callaghan A, Alvarado-Cardenas M, Marin A, et al. Statins and myositis: The role of anti-HMGCR antibodies. *Expert Rev Clin Immunol*. 2015;11(12):1277–1279.
7. Bohan A, Peter JB. Polymyositis and dermatomyositis (second of two parts). *N Engl J Med*. 1975;292(8):403–407.
8. Oddis CV, Reed AM, Aggarwal R, et al. RIM Study Group. Rituximab in the treatment of refractory adult and juvenile dermatomyositis and adult polymyositis: A randomised, placebo-phase trial. *Arthritis Rheum*. 2013;65(2):314–324.
9. Targoff IN, Mamyrova G, Trieu EP, et al. Childhood Myositis Heterogeneity Study Group; International Myositis Collaborative Study Group. A novel autoantibody to a 155-kd protein is associated with dermatomyositis. *Arthritis Rheum*. 2006;54(11):3682–3689.
10. Trallero-Araguas E, Rodrigo-Pendas JA, Selva-O'Callaghan A, et al. Usefulness of anti-p155 autoantibody for diagnosing cancer-associated dermatomyositis: A systematic review and meta-analysis. *Arthritis Rheum*. 2016;64:523–532.
11. Betteridge Z, McHugh N. Myositis-specific autoantibodies: An important tool to support diagnosis of myositis. *J Intern Med*. 2016;280(1):8–23.
12. Sato S, Kuwana M, Fujita T, Suzuki Y. Anti-CADM-140/MDA5 autoantibody titer correlates with disease activity and predicts disease outcome in patients with dermatomyositis and rapidly progressive interstitial lung disease. *Mod Rheumatol*. 2013;23:496–502.

CHAPTER 5

NEUROPHYSIOLOGY

Andria Merrison and Agyepong Oware

Nerve conduction studies (NCS) and electromyography (EMG) are used to aid the distinction between nerve, muscle and neuromuscular junction disorders. They are important diagnostic tests that must be considered within the context of the clinical picture and the results of other investigations. For some conditions, advances in genetics, imaging and serological tests have meant that neurophysiological tests may not be required.

DOI: 10.1201/9780429429323-5

NERVE CONDUCTION STUDIES (NCS)

Nerve conduction studies can be used to assess the functional and anatomical integrity of motor and sensory nerves. In routine clinical practice, the motor and sensory nerves in the distal lower and upper limbs are tested. These nerves are relatively superficial, and the stimulus intensity required is tolerable.

Motor nerve conduction studies involve supramaximal electrical stimulation at two or more sites along the length of the nerve. The evoked response is recorded from a muscle innervated by the nerve with a pair of surface electrodes, the active at the endplate region (the belly of the muscle) and the reference on the tendon. Supramaximal stimulation ensures the activation of all excitable axons. The stimulus is delivered at increasing distances from the muscle. The waveform produced, the compound muscle action potential (CMAP), is a sum of the muscle electrical activity at the vicinity of the active electrode. The latency, amplitude, duration and morphology of the CMAP at the different sites are analysed. The distances between the sites of stimulation and the latency differences are used to calculate conduction velocity.

Sensory conduction study involves supramaximal stimulation of sensory or mixed nerves with the recording electrodes being placed over the same nerve. The evoked response, (compound) sensory nerve action potential (SNAP), is a sum of the electrical activity from activated fibres. The attributes analysed are the latency, amplitude and conduction velocity. There are two methods for performing a sensory conduction study. Stimulation can be proximal (antidromic) or distal (orthodromic) to the recording electrode. The sensory conduction velocities are similar but antidromic stimulation produces higher amplitude SNAP than orthodromic stimulation. Sensory conduction studies assess the large myelinated axons only.

Routine NCS assesses the motor and sensory conduction velocities along the distal segments of the nerves, but the amplitudes of the action potentials reflect the integrity of the entire nerve. The latencies of the late responses, the H-reflex and F-wave, provide information about the conduction velocity along the proximal segments. The F-wave study is an extension of the motor conduction study and results from antidromic activation of motor neurons following stimulation of the nerve distally. The H-reflex is elicited by stimulating the tibial nerve in the popliteal fossa and recording at the soleus and median nerve at the elbow and recording at the flexor carpi radialis. The afferent limb of the reflex is sensory (spindle afferent) and the efferent is motor. The latencies of the late responses are height-dependent.

Nerve conduction studies can be used to:

- Localise weakness or sensory symptoms to the peripheral nervous system/lower motor neuron or the neuromuscular junction.

- Differentiate between axonal degeneration and demyelination as the underlying pathology. (The pattern of abnormalities helps differentiate between genetic/inherited and acquired demyelinating neuropathies.)
- Characterise the distribution of abnormalities – single nerve (mono-neuropathy, e.g., entrapment neuropathy), several nerves multi-focal or diffuse polyneuropathy, one or more nerve roots (radiculopathy), and plexus (plexopathy).
- Determine the type of fibres involved. Mixed sensory and motor, pure sensory/dorsal root ganglion or pure motor anterior horn cells (e.g., motor neurone disease, spinal muscular atrophy) are involved. Mixed sensory and motor involvement is the most common form of neuropathy.
- Identify subclinical neuropathies.
- Monitor peripheral nerve disorders.

Axonal degeneration (axonal neuropathy)

NCS
Low-amplitude SNAPs
Normal or reduced CMAPs
Normal conduction velocities

EMG
Spontaneous activity including fasciculations
Reduced number of motor units
Polyphasic, long-duration and high-amplitude motor unit action potentials

---

Demyelination (demyelinating neuropathy)

NCS
Slowing of conduction velocity
Conduction block
Dispersion of compound action potentials
Low-amplitude/absent SNAPs

EMG
Reduced recruitment
Spontaneous activity due to secondary axonal degeneration

Motor neuron disease (anterior horn cell dysfunction)

NCS
Normal sensory studies
Low-amplitude motor responses

EMG
Widespread denervation
Spontaneous activity
Fasciculations
Polyphasic, long-duration high-amplitude motor units
Reduced recruitment

Myopathy
NCS
Normal sensory and motor responses
EMG
Spontaneous activity (with or without)
Low-amplitude, polyphasic and short-duration motor unit action potentials
Early recruitment and full interference pattern

Limitations of NCS

Nerve conduction studies have a number of limitations:

- Electrical stimulation is painful. Some patients are unable to tolerate high enough stimulus intensity for supramaximal stimulation.
- Routine NCS does not assess small fibre function – thinly myelinated (Aδ) and unmyelinated fibres (C fibres).
- The sensory nerves in the proximal lower and upper limbs and the trunk are technically difficult to examine.
- The abnormalities are not disease-specific. This is mainly due to the limited repertoire of reactions to injury or disease in peripheral nerves. Most disease processes lead to axonal degeneration or demyelination.

Electromyography (EMG)

EMG is particularly helpful in identifying muscle disorders. It involves the insertion of a specialised needle containing a recording electrode into a muscle or range of muscles. EMG can be divided into four areas of analysis: insertional activity, spontaneous activity, motor unit potentials and interference pattern.

Insertion (or movement) of the EMG needle induces a burst of high-frequency potentials lasting a few hundred milliseconds. This is caused by mechanical stimulation or injury to muscle fibres. Decreased insertional activity occurs in fibrotic or severely atrophied muscle and periodic paralysis. Increased insertional activity is typically seen in denervation but may also be seen in other disorders, including inflammatory myopathies, myotonic disorders, acid maltase deficiency and hypothyroidism. Following the insertional activity, the normal muscle is "quiet" except when the needle is at the end plate.

In muscle or nerve disorders, the resting muscle shows abnormal spontaneous activity, which may take several forms:

Fibrillation potentials are spontaneous discharges (duration 1–5 milliseconds) arising from single muscle fibres (Figure 5.1). Positive sharp waves (comprising an initial positive spike followed by a slower negative potential) have a similar significance and often occur with fibrillation potentials. Both usually occur in denervation but are also seen in inflammatory myopathies, inclusion body myositis, muscle membrane instability, and endocrine and metabolic myopathies.

Fasciculation potentials are produced by the spontaneous discharge of muscle fibres of a whole motor unit. They are usually associated with motor neurone

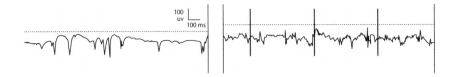

Figure 5.1 Positive sharp waves and fibrillation potentials.

disease, other peripheral nerve or root disorders, and may also be seen in thyro-toxic myopathy.

Complex repetitive discharges are prolonged bursts of high frequency (sounding like a machine gun) that are caused by near-synchronous repetitive firing of a group of muscle fibres. They are seen in neurogenic disorders (e.g., hereditary motor sensory neuropathy, spinal muscular atrophy) and myopathic disorders (inflammatory myopathy, muscular dystrophy, hypothyroidism and acid maltase deficiency).

Myotonic discharges are trains of electrical discharge that wax and wane in fre-quency and amplitude producing a characteristic "dive bomber" sound. They are seen in myotonic disorders (dystrophic and non-dystrophic, even in the absence of clinical myotonia), acid maltase deficiency, myopathy associated with choles-terol-lowering agents, periodic paralysis and hypothyroidism.

Myokymia

Repetitively firing single or multiple (grouped) motor units may be seen in demy-elinating conditions (CIDP, AIDP), radiation plexopathy and peripheral nerve hyperexcitability.

Motor unit potentials

A motor unit potential (MUP) is the summation of single-fibre potentials aris-ing within the same motor unit. It is recorded with an EMG electrode at both minimal and maximal activation of the muscle. The amplitude, duration, shape and recruitment pattern of MUPs are characteristics that are assessed and may provide further information about the nature of the disease (Figure 5.2).

The MUP amplitude depends on the number of fibres discharging close to the EMG needle. Therefore, MUP amplitude tends to be reduced in myopathic disor-ders due to the loss of functional muscle fibres.

In neurogenic disorders, MUP amplitudes are increased as collateral re-innerva-tion increases the number of fibres within a motor unit. The size of the electrical field of an individual muscle fibre is proportional to its diameter, so large MUPs may also be seen in conditions in which there is muscle hypertrophy (e.g., some muscular dystrophies).

MUP duration is a measure of the degree of synchrony of firing of fibres within a motor unit and is determined by the anatomical spread of the fibres within the unit, the length of muscle fibres, the speed of electrical propagation along the muscle fibres and membrane excitability. The duration is measured from the

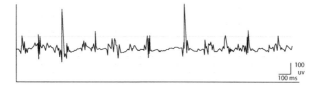

Figure 5.2 Myopathy low-amplitude, short-duration MUPs.

initial take-off to the return to baseline. It is prolonged in neurogenic disorders (with re-innervation and sprouting of axons) and reduced in myopathies due to loss of muscle fibres.

MUPs are usually bi- or tri-phasic. Phases are determined by the number of base-line crossings plus one. Polyphasic potentials arise when there is increased temporal dispersion of the firing of fibres within a motor unit. This may be seen in both neurogenic (e.g., motor neuropathies) and myogenic disorders (e.g., inflammatory myopathies).

Generally, MUPs have a fairly uniform shape and amplitude. Variability from moment to moment is referred to as instability and is usually seen in the context of jitter (see later). Instability occurs in neuromuscular junction disorders, in rapid denervation, in early re-innervation and in some inflammatory myopathies and inclusion body myositis.

Interference pattern

During increasing voluntary muscle contraction, the rate of individual motor unit firing increases and additional units become active (recruitment). A full interference pattern is seen when it is no longer possible to identify individual MUPs in the summated response.

In neurogenic disorders, the remaining motor neurons must fire faster than normal to achieve the same force. Even at maximum effort, individual MUPs can still be identified and the interference pattern is said to be reduced.

In myopathic disorders, the loss of muscle fibres means that a greater number of units need to be active to generate a given force. Therefore, a more complex interference pattern develops at a lower force of contraction (early recruitment). Neuromuscular junction disorders can also lead to early recruitment.

Repetitive nerve stimulation (RNS)

Repetitive supramaximal nerve stimulation at slow rates is usually at 3 Hz and measurement of the resulting muscle action potential is used to identify neuromuscular junction disorders. In myasthenia gravis, RNS demonstrates decrement: progressive reduction (>10%) of the CMAP amplitude/area from the first to fourth or fifth stimuli, followed by partial recovery. Decrement is also seen in Lambert–Eaton myasthenic syndrome at slow rates of stimulation (Figure 5.3). However, at higher rates (20 Hz) or following brief sustained contraction, the CMAP amplitude increases by over 100% (*facilitation*). Decrement may be seen in neurogenic disorders such as motor neuron disease.

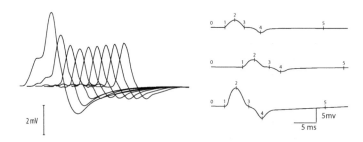

Figure 5.3 Decrement at 3Hz. Low-amplitude resting CMAP and 200% facilitation after brief exercise in Lambert–Eaton myasthenic syndrome (LEMS).

Single-fibre EMG and jitter

Single-fibre EMG can be used to detect activity from just a few muscle fibres within a motor unit. In this technique, the needle is positioned to record potentials from two muscle fibres, each innervated by a terminal branch of the same axon. In response to muscle contraction (or nerve stimulation), the two fibres will fire nearly simultaneously. The small time difference between the potentials is termed the interpotential interval and is a few tens of milliseconds. This interval reflects the neuromuscular transmission time between the two muscle fibres. The mean consecutive difference of successive interpotential intervals is called jitter.

The main source of jitter in normal nerve and muscle is the neuromuscular junction. Jitter is increased in neuromuscular junction disorders. Increased jitter may be seen in neuropathies with denervation and re-innervation and in myopathies associated with damage to the neuromuscular region. Jitter is reduced in muscular dystrophies and other myopathies that are associated with split muscle fibres.

Nerve conduction studies and EMG can be essential to establishing a diagnosis, including in situations where the clinical presentation is unclear or complex. Whilst relatively non-invasive, these tests are uncomfortable and may not be tolerated by all patients. Sedation may be required for these tests in young children. The tests may be technically difficult and inconclusive when there is significant oedema or excessive adipose tissue. There are no absolute contraindications, but a cautious approach is required with EMG in patients who are anticoagulated or have thrombocytopenia, and with NCS in patients with pacemakers and implanted cardiac defibrillators. Correct positioning of the electrodes and limb temperature are important. Ideally, the limb skin should be >32°C. The intensive care unit is a particularly challenging environment in which to undertake these tests due to the surrounding electrical noise.

Neurophysiology is a highly skilled area of medicine requiring close communication between the neurophysiologist and referring clinician. NCS and EMG abnormalities are not disease-specific. Therefore, careful consideration of the findings within the context of the patient's presentation is critical.

Further reading

Chichkova RI & Katzin L. (2010). EMG and nerve conduction studies in clinical practice. *Practical Neurology* 9(1):32–38.

Iwanami T et al. (2011). Decremental responses to RNS in motor neuron disease. *Clinical Neurophysiology* 122:2530–2536.

Kimura J. (2013). *Electrodiagnosis in Diseases of Nerve and Muscles: Principles and Practice*, 4th Edition, Oxford University Press, Oxford.

Mills K. (2016). *Oxford Textbook of Clinical Neurophysiology*, Oxford University Press, Oxford.

Rubin DI. (2021). *Clinical Neurophysiology*, Oxford University Press, Oxford.

Tim RW & Sanders DB. (1994). Repetitive nerve stimulation studies in the Lambert–Eaton myasthenic syndrome. *Muscle Nerve* 17:995–1001.

Whittaker RG. (2012). The fundamentals of electromyography. *Practical Neurology* 12(3):187–194.

CHAPTER 6

MUSCLE BIOPSY

Andria Merrison and Kathryn Urankar

Muscle biopsy has enabled the definition and diagnosis of muscle disease for decades and remains an invaluable diagnostic tool in assessing primary muscle disorders. Diagnosis depends on the skills of an expert pathologist working in collaboration with a specialist clinician. In this way, a multidisciplinary review of biopsies allows the setting of clinical context and careful analysis of biopsy findings, directing subsequent investigations and management strategies.

Muscle biopsies are not without inherent problems. Targeting the affected muscle is important in ensuring diagnostic material is sampled, although changes in severely affected muscle may mask the subtle changes required for diagnosis. Changes within muscle can also be very focal, both within and between muscles. For example, patchy changes in inflammatory muscle disease may be missed and require more than one biopsy for diagnosis. Interpretation of the changes seen in muscle may be difficult.

In some cases, myopathic changes may be secondary to another pathology. For example, inclusion body myositis may cause secondary mitochondrial changes and neurogenic disorders may show a range of secondary myopathic features. Necrosis can be seen in a wide range of different muscle disorders. Inflammatory changes in muscle may be primary (i.e. related to an underlying myositis) or an associated feature of a number of dystrophic conditions (e.g. Duchenne muscular dystrophy or some forms of limb girdle muscular dystrophy such as calpainopathy). Furthermore, certain pathological findings may be observed in different conditions and a variety of histological appearances may be seen in conditions associated with the same genetic variant. For example, ryanodine receptor 1 (RyR1) disorders can give rise to rods and/or cores, minicores, acute necrosis or fibre-type disproportion. Conversely, cores and rods are observed in association with variants in a host of other genes.

The genetic revolution has had an impact on the utility of muscle biopsy in the diagnosis of muscle disease. The rapidly developing application of next-generation sequencing has led to the analysis of panels of genes which enables a faster and more cost-effective diagnostic approach. Therefore, there are circumstances where advances in genetic testing have made muscle biopsy unnecessary. This is true for patients presenting with classical features of some muscular dystrophies, e.g. facioscapulohumeral muscular dystrophy, myotonic dystrophy and many of the limb girdle muscular dystrophies.

DOI: 10.1201/9780429429323-6

However, given the complex nature of some of the variants responsible for neuromuscular conditions, pathogenic variants may not be identified by routine genetic testing and may require the application of more specific techniques. Additionally, many new variants of uncertain significance are being uncovered through expansion in genetic testing and may require correlation with muscle biopsy to establish the pathogenicity of these novel variants. In some mitochondrial diseases, the responsible mitochondrial DNA mutation may only be found in muscle and therefore a muscle biopsy will be required for confirmatory genetic testing.

Despite all of these issues, muscle biopsy can be extremely useful. The context of the clinical picture remains essential in determining the diagnostic potential of muscle biopsy.

SAMPLING TECHNIQUE: OPEN AND NEEDLE BIOPSIES

Open muscle biopsies, usually carried out under local anaesthetic, allow direct visualisation of the muscle sampled and enable a larger, well-orientated and often less damaged sample to be submitted for analysis. This is the preferred method of sampling in adults. Needle biopsies (also performed with local anaesthetic) may allow for a more rapid acquisition of muscle and provide the opportunity to biopsy a range of muscles. This technique is often utilised in paediatric patients.

Open muscle biopsies are commonly carried out on vastus lateralis (quadriceps), gastrocnemius or deltoid muscles. Most is known about these muscles, and biopsies taken from other areas (e.g. distal or paraspinal muscles) may be more difficult to interpret.

Ideally, a muscle biopsy should be taken from an affected muscle that is mildly or moderately weak. In severely weak muscles, the microscopic appearances are often those of "end-stage muscle": muscle fibres are extensively atrophied and replaced by fat and connective tissue resulting in loss of specific diagnostic pathological features. Imaging, particularly magnetic resonance imaging (MRI), can be used in order to select an appropriate (affected) area of muscle for biopsy and may be particularly helpful in investigating patchy inflammatory muscle disease.

Once the sample has been taken, it is submitted fresh to the pathology laboratory in order to undergo a large range of histochemical, immunohistochemical and other testing. An initial sample is usually prepared for light microscopy where a panel of routine histological, histochemical and immunocytochemical stains can be applied. The specific tests performed depend on the diagnostic question and the initial pathology identified. Another sample of tissue is preserved in glutaraldehyde and can be submitted for electron microscopy. A third sample of tissue (if available) is frozen in liquid nitrogen for future biochemical and DNA analysis. Fresh tissue is required for testing in all cases, as fixation in formaldehyde destroys the activity of enzymes and affects analysis. Delays in transit to the laboratory can have similar effects. Immersion in water or saline may also distort some of the features observed.

Muscle histochemistry

Muscle is comprised of a combination of muscle fibres, nerves and blood vessels encased in a connective tissue sheath which protects the muscle from the effects of repeated contraction and relaxation. Muscle fibres are comprised of multiple myofibrils which themselves are composed of a series of sarcomeres, made up of interconnecting thin (actin) and thick (myosin) filaments. Contractions of muscle occur as a result of ATP-dependent movement of actin along the myosin filaments.

Enzyme histochemistry identifies two main fibre types: type 1 or slow-twitch fibres, and type 2 or fast-twitch fibres. Type 1 fibres have high oxidative and low glycolytic activity and are capable of generating force over a protracted period of time. In contrast, type 2 fibres have low oxidative and high glycolytic activity and are able to generate a large force rapidly. Type 2 fibres can be further subdivided into type 2A, 2B and 2C fibres, with the latter showing moderate rather than low oxidative activity. The different myofibre subtypes can be identified by staining with adenosine triphosphatase (ATPase) at different pHs. However, with the advent of immunohistochemistry, the use of antibodies against the myosin heavy chain isoforms is now more commonly utilised.

Motor nerve cell bodies originate in the anterior horn of the spinal cord. The neurone from the cell body branches to supply a variable number of muscle fibres (usually several hundred). The anterior horn cell, axon and the muscle fibres supplied constitute the motor unit. Muscle fibres from one motor unit are of a uniform type, and distributed in a limited area but randomly scattered and not clustered.

Most muscles in humans are of mixed fibre type, arranged in a checkerboard pattern. However, the proportion of each fibre type varies between muscles. Many factors can influence fibre type, including denervation, neuromuscular dysfunction, hormones, exercise, disuse, drugs and age (Table 6.1).

Histological stains

Haematoxylin and eosin (H&E) staining is the most important histological stain used in the interpretation of muscle biopsies. H&E stains highlight the overall structure of muscle tissue with muscle fibres appearing pink or eosinophilic, while nuclei appear blue. H&E stains enable the identification of a number of features, including myofibre size and variation, location of nuclei, the presence or absence of connective tissue (fibrosis and/or fat), necrotic fibres and/or basophilic degenerative/regenerative fibres, vacuoles, and inflammation. In addition, they allow for the assessment of blood vessels and nerves within the muscle. Rather than the presence of a single diagnostic feature, it is the combination of features within the context of the clinical setting that helps establish the diagnosis (Figure 6.1 and Figure 6.2).

Table 6.1 Muscle fibre types and histochemistry

	Type 1, Slow-twitch fibres	Type 2, fast-twitch fibres
ATPase	Dark at pH 4.5	Dark at pH 9.5
MATPase	Bright blue	2B violet, 2C light blue
PAS	Low glycogen content (pale)	High glycogen content (dark)
Oil Red O	High lipid content (red)	Low lipid content (pale)
NADH/SDH	High oxidative activity (dark)	Low oxidative activity (pale)
COX	High oxidative activity (dark)	Low oxidative activity (pale)
Phosphorylase	Low activity (paler)	High activity (darker)

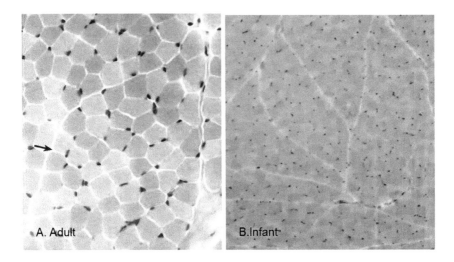

Figure 6.1 Normal muscle H&E 20x. (A) Adult muscle. (B) Infant muscle. These sections demonstrate the difference in myofibre diameters between the immature muscle of infants and children and the fully developed muscle of an adult.

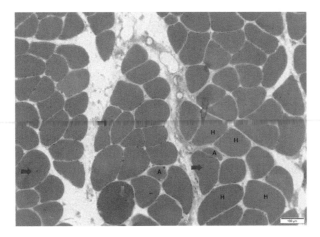

Figure 6.2 Myopathic muscle. H, hypertrophic myofibres; A, atrophic fibres. Green arrows highlight internal nuclei.

There are a number of patterns identifiable on routine H&E stains that can indicate a potential diagnosis and direct further studies. The classic features of a dystrophy include muscle fibre size variation, atrophy of myofibres, the presence of scattered necrotic fibres and/or basophilic degenerative/regenerative fibres, combined with an increase interstitial connective tissue. Split fibres are an additional feature identified in many limb girdle muscular dystrophies. A patchy inflammatory infiltrate may be seen in a number of dystrophies including Duchenne/ Becker muscular dystrophy, dysferlinopathies, calpainopathies and fasciohumeral muscular dystrophy (Figure 6.3).

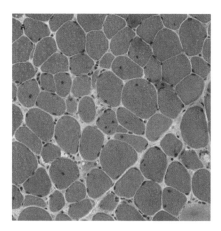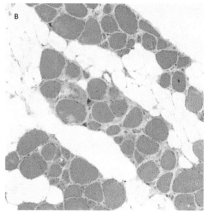

Figure 6.3 Dystrophic muscle. (A) Increased variation in myofibre dimeters, with frequent hypertrophic and atrophic fibres, combined with increased internal nuclei, increased endomysial connective tissue and occasional necrotic fibres (pale pink fibres). (B) More extensive changes with the replacement of muscle fibres by fat and connective tissue combined with further increased endomysial connective tissue.

The term "myopathy" is often used to describe more non-specific findings of muscle fibre size variation, type 1 fibre predominance and increased internal nuclei. Necrotic fibres and other various features may be seen but an increase in interstitial connective tissue is not characteristic.

The presence of group fibre atrophy, pyknotic nuclear clusters and fibre type grouping, alongside targets or targetoid fibres, point towards a neurogenic pathology (e.g. motor neurone disease, peripheral motor neuropathy). However, the changes seen may be subtle and non-specific and can depend on the duration and severity of denervation. Small angular fibres may form early in denervation, while in more chronic disorders, fibre type grouping may be seen (better demonstrated on MATPase, NADH or myosin staining). Fibre type grouping arises due to re-innervation by compensatory collaterals sprouting from the terminal axons of surviving neurons (Figure 6.4).

The presence of necrotic fibres and their distribution can be helpful in identifying the underlying aetiology, with groups of necrotic fibres seen in muscular dystrophies, perifascicular necrosis in antisynthetase disease, and isolated necrotic fibres in toxic or autoimmune aetiologies (i.e IMNM and in metabolic disorders. Vacuoles or "holes" within the muscle fibre vary in appearance and location within the muscle fibre, a feature which can also be used to point towards an underlying cause. However, correlation with material present within the vacuoles is typically required.

A panel of other histochemical stains is available to refine the diagnosis suspected based on the initial H&E findings (see Table 6.2). The modified Gömöri trichrome (GTC) stain is a very useful stain, enabling the identification of nuclei

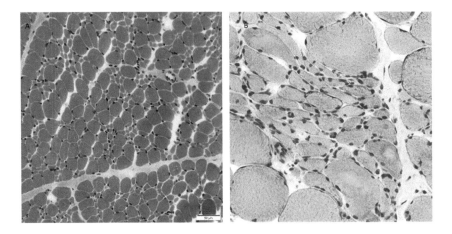

Figure 6.4 H&E muscle demonstrating group fibre atrophy on low power 10×
(A) and higher power (B) comprising clusters of small atrophic fibres.

including those of inflammatory cells (which stain bright red), muscle fibres
(which stain a blue-green colour), connective tissue (which stains a paler green),
myelin (which stains bright red) and mitochondria (which also stain bright red).
The accumulation of mitochondria within type 1 fibres and around the periphery of "ragged fibres" can be one of the characteristic features of mitochondrial
disorders. GTC staining can also identify other pathological features in muscle,
including nemaline rods, tubular aggregates, rimmed vacuoles and cytoplasmic
vacuoles, all of which stain red (Figure 6.5 and Figure 6.6).

Histochemical analysis of muscle also includes assessment of the storage of
energy sources within muscle. Periodic acid-Schiff (PAS staining) is utilised to
demonstrate both normal and abnormal storage of glycogen within myofibres;
the latter is normally observed in vacuoles in myofibres. Excess glycogen may
also be seen lying freely between myofibrils. It is most abundant in disorders
of the proximal end of the glycogenolytic/glycolytic pathway (e.g. debrancher
enzyme deficiency) but is usually absent in disorders of the distal end of the pathway. In acid maltase deficiency (Pompe disease), excess glycogen may be seen
within lysosomes (Figure 6.7).

Oil Red O or Sudan Black staining are utilised to demonstrate the lipid content
of muscle fibres. Type 1 fibres normally contain greater amounts of lipid compared to type 2 fibres, while this amount is increased in association with underlying lipid storage disorders. However, an increase in lipid storage may not be
identified in all cases. For example, in carnitine palmitoyltransferase deficiency
(CPT2 deficiency; the commonest cause of recurrent rhabdomyolysis in adults)
one may only see excess lipid in the muscle fibres immediately after an acute
episode (Figure 6.8).

Ragged Red Fibres in Mitochondrial Myopathy

A. H&E 40X granular fibre with peripheral enhancement.

B & C. Modified Gomori Trichrome 40X
    highlighting peripheral accumulation of
    mitochondria giving it a ragged red appearance.

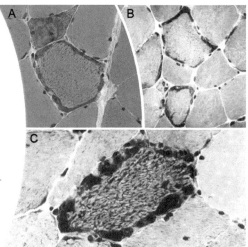

Figure 6.5 Ragged red fibres in mitochondrial myopathies. (A) H&E 40× granular fibres with peripheral enhancement of staining. (B and C) Modified Gömöri trichrome 40× highlighting the peripheral accumulation of mitochondria giving the fibres a "ragged red" appearance.

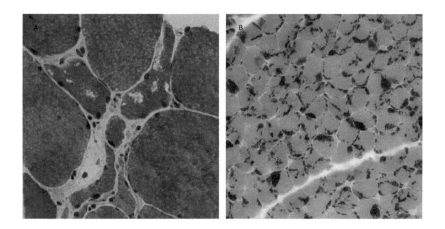

Figure 6.6 Modified Gömöri trichrome staining. (A) Rimmed vacuoles within myofibres. (B) The presence of numerous nemaline rods within myofibres.

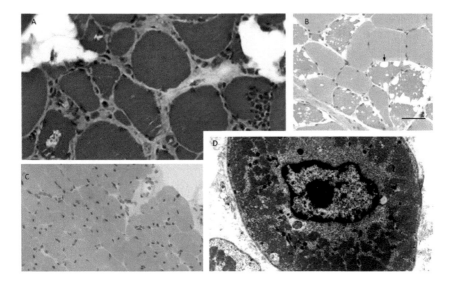

Figure 6.7 (A) H&E of muscle showing variation in myofibre diameters, increased connective tissue and invasion of intact fibres by inflammatory cells. (B) H&E showing subsarcolemmal vacuolation typical of glycogen storage disorders. (C) H&E showing increased internal nuclei characteristic of centronuclear myopathy. (D) Electron microscopy highlighting an internal nucleus.

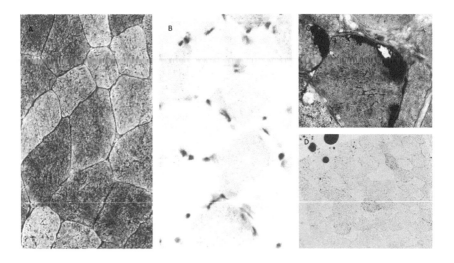

Figure 6.8 (A) PAS staining showing normal glycogen content in myofibres, with variation in content between type 1 and 2 fibres. (B) Normal Oil Red O staining showing normal lipid content in myofibres with variation in content between type 1 and 2 fibres. (C) PAS staining demonstrating accumulation of glycogen in a subsarcolemmal vacuole typical of a glycogen storage disorder. (D) Oil Red O staining showing increased lipid content in myofibres indicative of a lipid storage myopathy,

Histochemical techniques

Histochemical stains are used to demonstrate the biochemical properties of specific fibre types (and their selective involvement in disease). ATPase staining at different pHs can differentiate between type 1 (slow-twitch) and type 2 (fast-twitch) muscle fibres. However, immunostaining for myosin heavy chain fibre types is now more commonly performed. In normal muscle, there should be a chequerboard distribution of fibre types. This pattern may be lost in certain muscles, where a predominance of a particular fibre type may be normal (i.e. type 1 fibres in axial muscles and type 2 fibres in biceps and hamstrings). However, the pattern may also be lost in certain myopathies and in neurogenic disorders, where groupings of fibre types can be seen. Selective type 2 fibre atrophy is a non-specific finding reported in association with a variety of muscle problems, including disuse, ageing, paraneoplastic disorders and myasthenia gravis (Figure 6.9 and Figure 6.10).

Histochemical stains can also be useful in demonstrating the reduction or absence of an enzyme (e.g. phosphorylase in McArdle disease) or excess of a particular substrate (e.g. glycogen in glycogen storage disorders). They can also show structural changes in muscle that would not be evident with routine histological stains (e.g. cores in core myopathies or distribution of mitochondria).

Reduced nicotinamide adenine dinucleotide-tetrazolium reductase (NADH-TR), succinate dehydrogenase (SDH) and cytochrome c oxidase (COX) are the most useful oxidative enzymes studied in muscle. NADH-TR stains type 1 fibres a

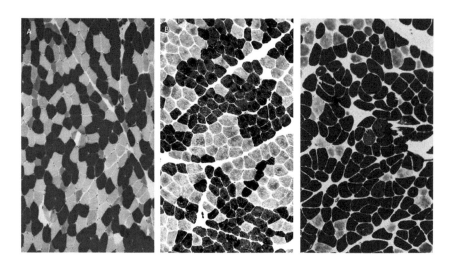

Figure 6.9 (A) MATPase histochemical staining showing relatively normal chequerboard distribution of myofibre types. Slow/type 1, dark blue; fast/type 2, light blue. (B) ATPase pH 4.5 showing grouping of myofibre types (dark, type 1; light, type 2) suggesting an underlying neurogenic disorder. (C) MATPase staining highlighting myopathic type grouping of type 1 fibres (dark blue) without associated grouping of type 1 fibres.

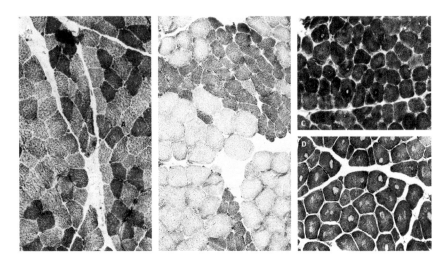

Figure 6.10 NADH histochemical staining. (A) A relatively normal chequerboard distribution of myofibre types. (B) Grouping of fibre types in a neurogenic disorder (dark fibres, type 1; light, type 2). (C) Targets within myofibres, showing a pale centre and a darkened rim. (D) Central cores showing pallor/loss of staining in myofibres.

darker blue than type 2 fibres (in contrast to myosin ATPase staining). It does not tend to stain the myofibrils but does stain the intermyofibrillar network (mitochondria and sarcoplasmic reticulum) and is therefore helpful in assessing the myofibrillar structure of myofibres. Cores, minicores and targets are best recognised on NADH staining. In addition, NADH staining can demonstrate the presence of lobulated fibres, moth-eaten fibres or ragged blue fibres (i.e. fibres with increased peripheral accumulation of mitochondria). Each of these findings can point towards specific underlying aetiologies.

SDH (blue) and COX (brown) are both mitochondrial stains and therefore also help distinguish fibre types (similar to NADHR), with type 1 fibres staining darker. COX staining in isolation helps identify COX-negative fibres which result from the impaired COX activity often seen in association with many types of mitochondrial disorders. However, combined staining for SDH and COX is most useful in the identification of COX-negative fibres, which appear blue rather than pale or negative.

There are a number of other histochemical stains which are useful in the diagnosis of muscle disorders. Congo red or crystal violet staining can help identify the deposition of amyloid in inclusion body myositis, while increased acid phosphatase staining can help confirm a diagnosis of Pompe disease. Alkaline phosphatase staining can highlight necrotic fibres and/or regenerating/immune myofibres, while positive staining for non-specific esterase can highlight denervated myofibres (see Table 6.2 and Table 6.3).

Table 6.2 Histological and histochemical stains

Stain	Use
H&E	Muscle fibre size and structure, nuclei, fibrosis, inflammation, nerves, blood vessels
NADH-TR	Muscle fibre type (type 1 fibres dark blue, type 2 light blue), mitochondrial distribution and abnormality; myofibrillar disruption including cores, targets, moth-eaten and lobulated fibres
SDH	Muscle fibre type (type 1 fibres dark brown, type 2 light brown), mitochondrial distribution and abnormality; myofibrillar disruption including cores, targets, moth-eaten and lobulated fibres
Myosin ATPase	Muscle fibre type (type 1 fibres light brown, type 2 dark brown) distribution
COX	Muscle fibre type, mitochondrial distribution and mitochondrial activity
Combined COX–SDH	Fibres with reduced/absent COX activity (some mitochondrial disorders) appear blue
PAS	Identifies excess glycogen (and other polysaccharides)
Oil Red O/Sudan Black	Lipid content (excess seen in lipid storage disorders, mitochondrial disorders) appears red on Oil Red O and black on Sudan Black
Congo red	Amyloid (present in sporadic and hereditary inclusion body myositis)
MHC class I (β2 microglobulin)	Upregulated expression in inflammatory muscle disease/primary myositis
Phosphorylase	Absent in McArdle disease (type V glycogenosis) and with other defects in glycogen synthesis; also identifies fibre type and cores (glycogen absence)
Phosphofructokinase	Absent in type VII glycogenosis; can be difficult to assess
Myoadenylate deaminase	Myoadenylate deaminase deficiency, tubular aggregates (dark); can be difficult to assess
Acid phosphatase	Raised in lysosomal storage disorders, type II glycogenosis, vacuolar myopathy and degenerating/necrotic fibres; very little is seen in normal muscle
Alkaline phosphatase	Raised in blood vessels (and other cell membranes where active transport occurs), some inflammatory myopathies and focal necrosis

(Continued)

Table 6.2 (Continued)   Histological and histochemical stains

Stain	Use
Menadione-linked α-glycerophosphate dehydrogenase	Acid maltase deficiency (Pompe disease); reduction of bodies and granular inclusions; accumulation of myofibrillar material in myofibrillar myopathies
Acetylcholinesterase	High acetylcholinesterase activity at neuromuscular junctions and some vacuoles

Abbreviations: H&E, haematoxylin and eosin; NADH-TR, reduced nicotinamide adenine dinucleotide-tetrazolium reductase; SDH, succinate dehydrogenase; COX, cytochrome c oxidase; PAS, periodic acid-Schiff; MHC, major histocompatibility complex.

Table 6.3   Histological stains

Stain	Use
H&E	Muscle fibre size and structure, nuclei, fibrosis, inflammation, nerves, blood vessels
NADH-TR	Muscle fibre type (type 1 fibres dark blue, type 2 light blue), mitochondrial distribution and abnormality, myofibrillar disruption, cores
SDH	Muscle fibre type (type 1 fibres dark brown, type 2 light brown), mitochondrial distribution and abnormality, cores
Myosin ATPase	Muscle fibre type (type 1 fibres light brown, type 2 dark brown) distribution
COX	Fibre type pattern, fibres with abnormal mitochondria or reduced mitochondrial activity, cores
Oil Red O	Lipid (intracellular): red
Sudan Black	Lipid and phospholipid: black

Abbreviations: H&E, haematoxylin and eosin; NADH-TR, reduced nicotinamide adenine dinucleotide-tetrazolium reductase; SDH, succinate dehydrogenase; COX, cytochrome c oxidase.

Immunohistochemistry

Antibodies directed against specific muscle proteins associated with the sarcolemmal contractile apparatus are routinely used as part of the assessment of muscle when an underlying dystrophic process is suspected. In general, when a pathogenic or disease-causing variant is present, there will be a loss of staining for the affected protein. For example, in Duchenne muscular dystrophy (DMD), there will be an absence of staining for dystrophin. In Becker muscular dystrophy (BMD), dystrophin staining may be reduced, patchy or focally lost but may also be normal. Secondary loss of sarcoglycan expression and increased dystrophin expression may also be observed in both DMD and BMD. However, advances in genetic testing have meant that in many suspected cases of muscular dystrophy, a muscle biopsy is not performed. There remains a utility for muscle biopsy in cases when a variant of unknown significance (VUS) is identified or a suspected variant is not detected. Demonstration of pathological changes in the muscle will help confirm the pathogenesis of the VUS and/or confirm the loss of the functional protein (Figure 6.11).

Immunohistochemical stains are of further utility in the diagnosis and classification of forms of myositis. Immunostaining is used to determine the types of inflammatory cells present, including lymphocytes (T and B cells) and macrophages. Upregulation of other inflammatory markers is usually seen, in particular upregulation of major histocompatibility complex (MHC) class II (i.e. β-2 microglobulin).

The characteristic feature of inflammatory myopathies is the presence of inflammatory infiltrates, mainly lymphocytes and some macrophages. Upregulation of MHC class I molecules may also be seen. More recently, the pattern of upregulation of MHC class II, expression of MXA (human myxovirus resistance protein A) and expression of type 1 interferon has been used to subclassify types of primary myositis.

In dermatomyositis, the inflammatory infiltrates tend to be perivascular and are mainly comprised of helper T-cells (T4+, CD4). Isolated necrotic fibres or groups of fibres (due to infarction) and perifascicular atrophy may also be seen. These fibres often express membrane attack complex (MAC or C5b9), which can also be expressed in capillaries. While MHC class I expression is seen, often with a peripheral gradient of staining, there is an absence of expression of MHC class II. Sarcoplasmic MXA expression is observed.

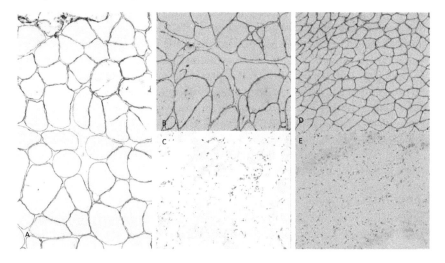

Figure 6.11 Immunohistochemical staining of muscles for the dystrophic-associated protein. (A) Retained "normal" sarcolemmal staining for DAPs, although variation in myofibre diameters is noted combined with occasional split (invaginated) fibres. (B) Retained normal staining for dystrophin compared to (C) complete loss of staining for dystrophin in Duchenne muscular dystrophy. (D) Normal staining for merosin in unaffected muscle compared to (E) complete loss of sarcolemmal staining for merosin in merosin-deficient LGMD.

Muscle diseases

Antisynthetase syndrome is characterised by perifascicular necrosis rather than atrophy and CD138-positive plasma cells may be present as part of the inflammatory infiltrate. Upregulation of both MHC class I and class II is characteristic and there is the absence of the type 1 interferon signature.

In contrast, inclusion body myositis inflammatory infiltrates tend to be scattered within the endomysium of fascicles, with cytotoxic T-cells (T8+, CD8) making up the majority of infiltrating cells. Partial invasion of muscle fibres is common (i.e. clusters of inflammatory cells apparently compressing or indenting non-necrotic muscle fibres) and necrotic fibres can be seen scattered throughout the fascicles. In inclusion body myositis, there will be a generalised upregulation of MHC class I without expression of MHC class II. MAC expression may be seen on some necrotic fibres but is not observed on capillaries. The classic diagnostic feature is the identification of p62 positive granular subsarcolemmal inclusions within rimmed vacuoles. These can also stain with TDP-43, LC3 and ubiquitin. Concomitant mitochondrial abnormalities are characteristic.

Immune-mediated necrotising myopathies tend to show a paucity of inflammation within the muscle and instead demonstrate the presence of scattered necrotic fibres. The necrotic fibres tend to show sarcoplasmic expression of MAC (C5b9) and a characteristic pattern of diffuse sarcoplasmic staining for p62. MHC class I may be upregulated, but MHC class II expression is never observed.

Electron microscopy
Although considered to be an outdated modality in other fields, electron microscopy (EM) remains extremely helpful in the diagnosis of muscle disorders. EM allows for visualisation of the ultrastructure of muscle, can identify distortions in muscle structure and the presence of characteristic inclusions, and can confirm the nature of a range of structural abnormalities which characterise many of the common congenital myopathies. EM is particularly useful in identifying abnormal mitochondria and characteristic paracrystalline inclusions in mitochondria, confirming an underlying mitochondrial myopathy prior to enzymatic or genetic testing. It can also demonstrate the presence of other characteristic inclusions such as rods in nemaline myopathy, glycogen within vacuoles in the various glycogen storage disorders, and the tubulofilamentous inclusions often present in inclusion body myositis or oculopharyngeal muscular dystrophy.

Congenital myopathies
Congenital myopathies are a diverse group of disorders that may demonstrate a variety of features on muscle biopsy, including ultrastructural abnormalities. In some forms, the muscle fibre architecture is disrupted (e.g. central core disease, multicore or centronuclear myopathy) and nuclei may be displaced from the periphery to the centre of muscle fibres (e.g. centronuclear myopathy). In other types of congenital myopathy, particular proteins form abnormal structures or accumulations (e.g. nemaline myopathy, myofibrillar myopathy) or demonstrate abnormality within organelles (e.g. tubular aggregate myopathy). Depending on the subtype, these changes can be identified on routine H&E stains or on particular histochemical and/or immunohistochemical stains.

Further reading

Dubowitz V, Sewry CA & Oldfors A. (2021). *Muscle biopsy: A Practical Approach*. 5th edn. London: Saunders Elsevier.

Merve A, Schneider U, Kara E, Papadopoulou C & Stenzel W. (2022). Muscle biopsy in myositis: What the rheumatologist needs to know. *Best Practice Research Clinical Rheumatology* 36(2):101763.

CHAPTER 7

MUSCLE IMAGING

Rajat Chowdhury

Muscle imaging studies can provide an increased understanding of neuromuscular disease patterns, as well as their activity, severity and distribution, to help provide answers to diagnostic challenges. In addition, imaging studies are often used to support clinical and laboratory findings. Magnetic resonance imaging (MRI) is helpful in evaluating specific areas of muscle oedema and areas of replacement of muscle tissue by fat, muscle volume loss or increase; as well as identifying which muscles are involved and which geographical territory within the affected muscles the changes are affecting. MRI is both sensitive and specific in the diagnosis of many neuromuscular diseases, particularly in the diagnosis of inherited myopathies, which have certain typical and/or characteristic patterns of muscle involvement or sparing which can be visualised on MRI. For example, in most cases of ryanodine receptor 1 (*RYR1*) myopathy, the vastus muscles are affected more than the rectus femoris muscle in the thigh, and the soleus muscle is more affected than the medial and lateral gastrocnemius muscles in the posterior calf. MRI can also help identify appropriate targets for muscle biopsy.

Muscle MRI is also helpful in evaluating inflammatory myopathies not only for diagnosis with certain characteristic patterns relating to specific inflammatory myopathies but also for monitoring progress and response to treatment. Most inflammatory myopathies demonstrate diffuse inflammatory fluid in the affected muscles, as evidenced by T2 signal hyperintensity, with the exception of inclusion body myositis (IBM), where there is an overriding asymmetric pattern of fatty infiltration within the affected muscles.

Computed tomography (CT) is sensitive in detecting the replacement of muscle tissue with fat and reduction in muscle volume, particularly in advanced or chronic neuromuscular disease. It may also be used if MRI is contraindicated, although early disease is usually difficult to identify on CT (Figure 7.1).

Ultrasound examination can be helpful in detecting fluid and oedema in the soft tissues as well as in the identification of the replacement of muscle tissue with fat. Ultrasound is often used to guide radiological muscle biopsies.

Dystrophinopathies, such as Duchenne muscular dystrophy, are seen to preferentially affect the gluteal and adductor magnus muscle in the thigh and the gastrocnemius and peroneus longus muscle in the calf on MRI scans. Limb girdle muscular dystrophies, in contrast, are seen to preferentially affect the posterior thigh muscles in addition to the gluteal and adductor muscles. The muscles least affected include the gracilis, sartorius and tibialis posterior muscles (Figure 7.2 and Figure 7.3).

DOI: 10.1201/9780429429323-7

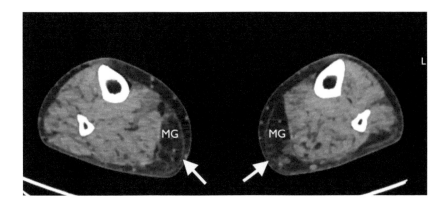

Figure 7.1 The distinctive and characteristic CT pattern of replacement of muscle tissue with fat in the medial gastrocnemius muscles bilaterally in the case of IBM. MG, medial gastrocnemius.

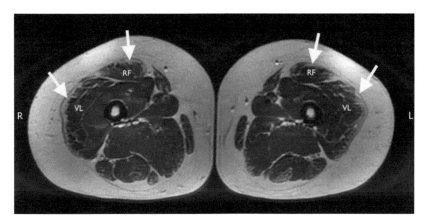

Figure 7.2 The distinctive and characteristic MRI pattern of muscle involvement in collagen VI-related myopathies, which target the periphery of the vastus muscles and gastrocnemius muscles. VL, vastus lateralis; RF, rectus femoris.

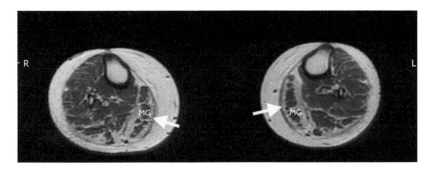

Figure 7.3 The distinctive and characteristic MRI pattern of muscle involvement in collagen VI-related myopathies, which target the periphery of the vastus muscles and gastrocnemius muscles. MG, medial gastrocnemius.

Muscle MRI protocols for neuromuscular disease should include both fat-sensitive (T1-weighted) and fluid-sensitive sequences (T2-weighted). The fluid-sensitive sequences should be performed with fat saturation (FS), usually STIR (short-tau inversion recovery), T2 or proton density (PD), to allow accurate evaluation of fat and fluid distribution within muscle. These sequences should be performed in multiple planes (usually coronal and axial). In general, muscle oedema is identified by signal hyperintensity on STIR, T2FS and PDFS sequences, and fatty tissue replacement is identified by signal hyperintensity on T1-weighted sequences (Figure 7.4 and Figure 7.5). The key diagnostic patterns are assessed from the axial series of the lower limbs which is usually of high diagnostic yield but whole-body MRI can often give a more specific analysis with regard to which muscles are preferentially affected and which are preferentially spared. This can be particularly useful in diagnosing hereditary myopathies. In more advanced

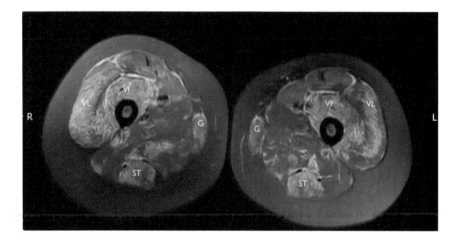

Figure 7.4 An inflammatory myopathy with diffuse T2 signal hyperintensity in the thigh muscles, especially in vastus lateralis (VL), vastus intermedius (VI), gracilis (G) and semitendinosus (ST), along with inflammatory fluid tracking along the anterior and intermuscular fasciae, more so on the right.

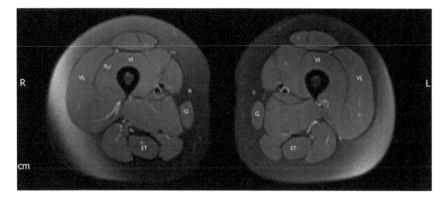

Figure 7.5 Complete resolution of Figure 7.4 with glucocorticoid treatment.

diseases, however, muscle involvement can be far more widespread and thus diagnostically less helpful.

The differential diagnosis of inflammatory muscle signals on MRI is wide and includes polymyositis, dermatomyositis, drug toxicity, infection and rhabdomyolysis. The differential diagnosis of fat infiltration in muscle on MRI includes denervation and neuropathy, disuse and previous trauma. Interpretation of muscle MRI is therefore dependent on the clinical context, which will then predetermine its value in guiding related diagnostic and management pathways.

CHAPTER 8

GENETIC INVESTIGATIONS IN NEUROMUSCULAR DISEASES

Kate Sergeant and Carl Fratter

INTRODUCTION

Genetic investigations play an important role in the diagnosis of suspected neuromuscular disease. Establishing a genetic diagnosis provides information regarding prognosis and risks to other family members and allows advice to be given in relation to reproductive options. Moreover, genetic testing increasingly allows for the possibility of targeted treatments and the potential for inclusion in clinical trials. The "genomic revolution" has led to genetic investigations increasingly becoming a first-line investigation in the diagnosis of neuromuscular disease. Historically, a muscle biopsy was often performed early in the diagnostic pathway, and results of muscle histology and biochemical analyses would then guide genetic testing, which was typically limited to testing for common pathogenic variants or sequencing of individual genes known to be involved in the suspected conditions. The development of next-generation sequencing (NGS) and other technological advances has enabled timely and cost-effective genetic testing of blood DNA with a high diagnostic yield (Herman et al., 2021). Therefore, muscle biopsy may now only be necessary in more limited circumstances, such as when genetic testing has not led to a diagnosis or when genetic testing has detected variants of uncertain clinical significance.

Currently, a number of genetic testing strategies and approaches may be employed depending on the suspected neuromuscular disorder and the resources available to genetic testing laboratories. These include simple low-cost targeted tests (e.g., copy number variant detection for dystrophinopathies or testing for the repeat expansions associated with myotonic dystrophy) as well as more comprehensive NGS approaches such as whole-exome sequencing (WES) and whole-genome sequencing (WGS).

For consideration of appropriate genetic testing methods, neuromuscular disorders can be grouped by their genetic characteristics. The subsequent sections summarise these characteristics and outline appropriate testing strategies, based on current approaches in the United Kingdom and in many other centres/countries worldwide. This is followed by a discussion of the limitations of genetic testing.

DOI: 10.1201/9780429429323-8

Dystrophinopathies

Duchenne muscular dystrophy (DMD) and Becker muscular dystrophy (BMD) are caused by pathogenic variants in the X-linked *DMD* gene. This gene encodes dystrophin, the largest gene in the human genome. The majority of causative variants are large deletions or duplications of one or more exons. Therefore, initial genetic analysis is often limited to testing for exon-level copy number variants (CNVs) using targeted methods such as multiplex ligation-dependent probe amplification (MLPA) analysis. If a causative deletion or duplication is not identified, then sequence analysis of the coding regions of the *DMD* gene can be carried out to detect small nucleotide variants (SNVs), such as missense or nonsense changes. More detailed information regarding genetic analysis for DMD and BMD can be found in "EMQN Best Practice Guidelines for Genetic Testing in Dystrophinopathies" (Fratter et al., 2020).

Short tandem repeat expansion disorders

Some neuromuscular diseases are caused by expansion of short tandem repeats (STRs) and these often require more specialised testing techniques. Expansions are typically categorised into ranges for normal, intermediate and pathogenic numbers of repeats. Due to the large size of some pathogenic expansions and the nature of the repetitive sequence, they can be refractory to standard polymerase chain reaction (PCR) amplification and may be missed by short-read NGS and bioinformatic analysis pipelines, which are usually optimised for calling smaller sequence variants.

Myotonic dystrophy type I (DM1) and type II (DM2) are caused by monoallelic expansion of repeats in the non-coding regions of the *DMPK* (CTG) and *CNBP* (CCTG) genes, respectively. Each disorder can be excluded by the presence of two alleles within the normal repeat size range at the particular locus. This can be detected by conventional PCR across the repeat region followed by sizing of the amplification products, typically by fluorescent capillary electrophoresis. If only one allele in the normal range is detected, then further investigation using repeat-primed PCR and/or Southern blotting analysis is necessary to differentiate between homozygosity for a normal-sized allele and an expansion in the affected range. WGS technologies may be used to detect repeat expansions if there is no PCR step in the initial library preparation, which avoids preferential amplification of the shorter fragments. Specialised bioinformatic data analysis tools can then be employed to interrogate the WGS data to identify repeat expansions. Using WGS to detect repeat expansions allows for alternative diagnoses to be interrogated at the same time (see later).

Similarly, oculopharyngeal muscular dystrophy (OPMD) is almost exclusively caused by expansion of a GCN (where N can be any nucleotide) repeat, encoding the amino acid alanine, in exon 1 of the *PABPN1* gene. However, in OPMD, the largest expansions consist of only 17 GCN repeats and so are readily detected by a simple PCR and sizing assay, as well as being detectable by WGS and most other NGS methods.

Facioscapulohumeral muscular dystrophy

Facioscapulohumeral muscular dystrophy (FSHD) is caused by very unusual genetic mechanisms; these differ between FSHD type 1 (FSHD1) and FSHD type 2 (FSHD2) but ultimately lead to the relaxation of chromatin in the subtelomeric region of the q arm of chromosome 4 (4q) and hence expression of the *DUX4* gene.

FSHD1 is caused by contraction (partial deletion) of the 3.3kb D4Z4 subtelomeric repeats on chromosome 4q. The contraction also has to be on a "permissive" haplotype in order to be associated with disease. A very similar repeat region is present on chromosome 10, but this is not associated with disease. Testing is typically carried out by Southern blotting to size the D4Z4 repeat region using restriction enzymes to distinguish between repeats on chromosomes 4 and 10. Haplotype analysis can also be carried out to determine if contracted D4Z4 repeats are present on a permissive background.

FSHD2 is caused by hypomethylation of the D4Z4 repeats and most cases of hypomethylation result from a pathogenic sequence variant in the *SMCHD1* gene. If there are clinical features typical of FSHD but initial analysis has not identified a contracted D4Z4 repeat on chromosome 4 (but has identified at least one permissive haplotype), then methylation studies for FSHD2 should be considered, typically undertaken by bisulphite conversion of genomic DNA (to convert unmethylated cytosine to uracil) and subsequent sequencing. Finally, sequence analysis of *SMCHD1* can be carried out in order to identity a pathogenic variant if hypomethylation is detected.

Genetically heterogeneous neuromuscular disorders

For groups of disorders with considerable genetic heterogeneity, such as limb girdle muscular dystrophies (LGMD) or congenital myasthenic syndromes (CMS), a wider approach to genetic analysis is generally more effective. Panels of genes (for example, those curated in PanelApp, https://panelapp.genomicsengland.co .uk/) can be sequenced simultaneously using targeted NGS technologies or a virtual panel can be applied to exome or genome data. Gene agnostic exome or genome analysis may be more useful where there is a much wider differential diagnosis, but it usually requires sequencing of multiple family members, such as a parent–child trio for paediatric patients without a family history.

Analysis of sequencing data for SNVs is typically restricted to coding regions plus splice sites. To maximise sensitivity, analysis should also aim to detect CNVs for relevant genes. This can be achieved by additional techniques such as MLPA or microarray or ideally by including bioinformatics CNV tools in the NGS data analysis pipeline.

In contrast to the targeted techniques described earlier, more extensive analysis comes with the task of interpreting the many sequence variants that will be identified. Variants of uncertain significance (VUSs) are often identified and determining their likelihood of clinical significance is challenging (see "Limitations" section). Laboratories may choose not to report VUSs in order to minimise misinterpretation of such findings. Furthermore, the chance of incidental findings is increased with wider analyses, such as detecting carrier status for an unrelated recessive disorder or identifying a pathogenic variant in a gene associated with cancer susceptibility. Disclosing such incidental findings may be subject to local policy and guidelines (e.g., Green et al., 2013, and subsequent updates).

Mitochondrial disorders

Mitochondrial disorders have significant genetic heterogeneity and so are amenable to the NGS approaches outlined thus far. However, mitochondrial disorders can be caused by pathogenic variants in either nuclear or mitochondrial DNA (mtDNA)-encoded genes and are further complicated by heteroplasmy of the multicopy mtDNA. Therefore, a single NGS assay for comprehensive mitochondrial genetic testing is not routinely available in most centres, although WGS is increasingly being developed for this purpose.

The mitochondrial genome is a small (16.6kb) circular molecule which is strictly maternally inherited and is present in multiple (100–1000s) copies per cell. Pathogenic mtDNA variants are typically heteroplasmic (i.e., a mixture of wild-type molecules and molecules containing the variant are present). Levels of heteroplasmy can vary between tissues and over time; importantly, variants may be at very low levels (<5%) or absent in blood from adults and older children. Therefore, muscle is often preferred for mtDNA analysis, especially in adults. When muscle is not available, urine can be a useful alternative. Laboratory methods that are able to detect low levels of variant (down to ~5%) and that can accurately quantify heteroplasmy are preferred. Targeted analysis for common pathogenic mtDNA variants, such as m.3243A>G and large-scale mtDNA deletions, may be adopted as a first-line test, particularly if the phenotype is suggestive of a specific variant. NGS of the whole mitochondrial genome requires high read depth to achieve a sufficiently low limit of heteroplasmy detection, and can be used as a first-line test or following targeted testing if necessary. "Genetic Testing for Mitochondrial Disease: The United Kingdom Best Practice Guidelines" (Mavraki et al., 2023) can be referred to for further details.

Limitations and further analysis

Despite the genomic revolution, significant limitations of genetic (or genomic) testing remain.

Laboratory turnaround times are highly variable and typically it can take weeks or months for a result, particularly due to the complexity of both laboratory wet work and analysis. Even when testing is requested urgently, turnaround times are likely to be several days for more simple tests or several weeks for NGS-based tests.

Although genetic tests for a few disorders, such as DM1 and DM2, approach 100% sensitivity, in general failure to identify a genetic cause does not exclude a genetic diagnosis. This is due to technical and analytical limitations as well as the possibility of other, as yet unknown, genes associated with the specific neuromuscular phenotype. Moreover, when a genetic diagnosis is made, this is typically definitive, but there may be uncertainty regarding prognosis.

The limitations in test sensitivity are most pronounced for neuromuscular disorders with high genetic heterogeneity. The sensitivity of NGS approaches, including WES and WGS, is affected by incomplete sequence coverage, restricting analysis to specific regions (such as coding exons plus splice sites) and the inability to interpret the pathogenicity and clinical significance of all variants detected.

Although the development of guidelines for variant classification (Richards et al., 2015; ClinGen Sequence Variant Interpretation, https://clinicalgenome.org /working-groups/sequence-variant-interpretation/) has helped standardise approaches, variant interpretation remains challenging.

Multidisciplinary teams (MDTs) can be helpful in evaluating the clinical significance of VUSs, but in many cases this remains uncertain and further studies are required to try to confirm or exclude the putative genetic diagnosis.

If patients remain undiagnosed, because either no candidate causative variants were identified or VUSs were identified, then there may be options for additional analysis. In some cases, other "routine" diagnostic investigations, such as muscle biopsy or muscle imaging, may be sufficient to reclassify a VUS as (likely) pathogenic. More often, functional studies, other "omics" (such as transcriptomics and proteomics) and/or emerging genomics (such as long-read NGS and optical genome mapping) would be required to further pursue a possible genetic diagnosis. These are not available in most diagnostic settings, although collaboration with research groups may be possible. For further discussion, see Wortmann et al. (2022).

Conclusion

In summary, there are many different genetic tests available to investigate suspected neuromuscular disease and these have become more comprehensive with recent developments in sequencing technologies enabling genome-wide data to be interrogated in a single test. However, it is important to consider that even if exome or genome sequencing has been performed, more specialised testing may be required to diagnose certain disorders such as FSHD or mtDNA disease. Furthermore, if patients remain undiagnosed after the aforementioned testing strategies, this does not exclude a genetic diagnosis and there may be options for follow-up studies.

Further reading

Fratter et al., 2020, *Eur J Hum Genet.* 28(9):1141–1159. PMID: 32424326
Green et al., 2013, *Genet Med.* 15(7):565–574. PMID: 23788249
Herman et al., 2021, *Muscle Nerve.* 63(3):304–310. PMID: 33146414
Mavraki et al., 2023, *Eur J Hum Genet.* 31(2):148–163. PMID: 36513735
Richards et al., 2015, *Genet Med.* 17(5):405–424. PMID: 25741868
Wortmann et al., 2022, *J Inherit Metab Dis.* 45(4):663–681. PMID: 35506430

CHAPTER 9

MANAGEMENT, TREATMENT AND THERAPY FOR NEUROMUSCULAR CONDITIONS

Andria Merrison

Managing people living with neuromuscular conditions requires a holistic, dedicated and collaborative multidisciplinary team. We are entering a new era where specific disease-modifying or curative treatments are increasingly available for conditions previously considered unremittingly progressive. The number of such treatments is growing, particularly with the expansion in understanding of genetics and gene-modifying agents, such that there are several options for people living with Duchenne muscular dystrophy or spinal muscular atrophy. However, for many patients, the approach is one of managing symptoms, minimising comorbidity and providing supportive therapies (Table 9.1).

Successful management is likely to require medical input across a range of disciplines (neurologists, respiratory physicians, cardiologists, geneticists, rehabilitation physicians, palliative medicine physicians, psychologists, endocrinologists, rheumatologists, anaesthetists, spinal surgeons, pathologists and neurophysiologists). The multidisciplinary team will also include physiotherapists, occupational therapists, speech and language therapists, orthotists, and social workers. This is likely to require working across a range of organisations in health, social care and community settings.

DOI: 10.1201/9780429429323-9

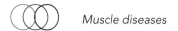

Table 9.1 Specific treatments for muscle diseases

Condition	Treatment
Duchenne muscular dystrophy	Steroids (glucocorticoids) in childhood, gene therapy: ataluren (nonsense mutations), eteplirsen (exon 51 skippable mutations), viltolarsen and golodirsen (exon 53 skippable mutations), casimersen (exon 45 skippable mutations)
Myotonic dystrophy	Modafinil for sleepiness, mexiletine for myotonia
Polymyositis/dermatomyositis	Steroids, azathioprine, methotrexate, mycophenolate, cyclophosphamide, IVIg, plasma exchange
Spinal muscular atrophy	Gene modifying therapy: nusinersen (intrathecal injection) and risdiplam (oral medication)
Paramyotonia congenita	Mexiletine, acetazolamide
Myotonia congenita	Mexiletine
Hyperkalaemic periodic paralysis	Acute: salbutamol Prevention: acetazolamide, thiazide diuretics
Hypokalaemic periodic paralysis	Acute: K^+ supplements Prevention: low Na^+-high K^+ diet, acetazolamide, spironolactone
Anderson–Tawil syndrome	K^+ management, acetazolamide, implantable defibrillator
Malignant hyperthermia	Dantrolene, treat hyperkalaemia and arrhythmias, sodium bicarbonate for acidosis
Mitochondrial disease	Co-enzyme Q10
β-oxidation defects	Avoid fasting, diet: low fat, sufficient carbohydrates
Primary carnitine deficiency	Carnitine supplements
Long chain acyl dehydrogenase deficiency	Diet: carbohydrate, medium chain triglycerides and reduced long-chain fatty acids
Multiple acyl-coA dehydrogenase deficiency/riboflavin deficiency	Riboflavin supplements
Acid maltase deficiency (Pompe disease)	Enzyme replacement therapy: α-glucosidase, avalglucosidase alfa

INFLAMMATORY MUSCLE DISEASE

Corticosteroids are the first-line agents used in inflammatory muscle disorders (including polymyositis and dermatomyositis). If longer-term treatment is required, steroid-sparing agents, including methotrexate, azathioprine or mycophenolate, may be used. In patients with connective tissue disorders, cyclophosphamide or rituximab may be considered. Intravenous immunoglobulin (or plasma exchange) may be used in the acute setting, particularly in severe dermatomyositis.

Myotonic dystrophy

Modafinil may be helpful in treating excessive daytime sleepiness and mexiletine may alleviate myotonia. Treatment may also be required for the multisystem complications of myotonic dystrophy (DM). Gene therapy, including the development of antisense molecules that will reduce mutant DPMK (the myotonic dystrophy protein kinase gene that causes this condition), offers potential hope for disease-modifying therapies in DM1.

Duchenne muscular dystrophy

Corticosteroids form the mainstay of treatment in childhood. There is evidence that they delay the onset of loss of ambulation, preserve respiratory function and reduce the need for scoliosis surgery. There is less evidence for ongoing benefit in adulthood. Gene therapy is developed rapidly in treating people living with Duchenne muscular dystrophy (DMD) and a number of mutation-specific treatments have regulatory approval. These include ataluren (nonsense mutations), eteplirsen (exon 51 skippable mutations), viltolarsen and golodirsen (exon 53 skippable mutations), and casimersen (exon 45 skippable mutations) but they are not universally available.

Spinal muscular atrophy

There are two licensed gene-modifying therapies for spinal muscular atrophy (SMA): nusinersen (intrathecal injections) and risdiplam (an oral medication). These treatments have had excellent early outcomes; with respect to improved muscle strength in the limbs, trunk and respiratory muscle function for babies and children presenting with SMA. Their efficacy longer term and for patients presenting in adult life are being assessed. Further gene replacement therapy trials are underway, including onasemnogene abeparvovec. In addition, oral salbutamol has been used and reported to improve muscle strength in some patients.

Glycogen storage disease (Pompe disease)

Enzyme replacement therapy (glucosidase α) is licensed for Pompe disease and has been used very effectively since 2006. Avalglucosidase alfa-ngpt is a synthetic oligosaccharide, available since 2021, which may have increased efficacy in reducing the accumulation of glycogen. The first patients treated with enzyme replacement therapy in infancy are now surviving into adulthood.

Gene-modifying therapy provides an attractive future way of treating patients with Pompe disease, tackling the problems of multisystem disease and the central nervous system. A number of approaches, including recombinant adenovirus and lentivirus vectors, are being explored.

Channelopathies

Periodic paralysis can be alleviated with potassium normalisation and acetazolamide. Mexiletine is used for myotonia in myotonia congenita and in some patients with myotonic dystrophy too.

Mitochondrial disease

Some patients report improvement in functional strength and reduced fatigue when taking regular coenzyme Q10.

Respiratory complications

A number of muscle conditions are associated with respiratory complications (see Table 9.2), usually respiratory muscle (diaphragmatic and intercostals) weakness. Respiratory surveillance (lung function tests, overnight oximetry and carbon dioxide monitoring) is required for these patients. Early respiratory weakness is often detected at night, causing sleep disruption, early morning headaches, daytime somnolence/fatigue, loss of appetite and cognitive difficulties.

Non-invasive ventilation, bilevel positive airway pressure (BiPAP), is usually the treatment of choice. In some circumstances, including later in disease progression, tracheostomy ventilation may be an option that is considered. A growing number of people living with Duchenne muscular dystrophy and other muscle conditions use tracheostomies and portable ventilation units.

In some conditions, such as myotonic dystrophy, early upper airway weakness may lead to obstructive sleep apnoea. Some of these patients will benefit from continuous positive airway pressure (CPAP) ventilation. A relatively small number of patients (including some patients with myotonic dystrophy) will also have centrally driven breathing problems, including central apnoea, which will require ventilation set to trigger supportive ventilation when such problems arise.

Many patients, particularly those with significant bulbar involvement, will need support with cough management. This can include respiratory physiotherapy techniques such as breath stacking and for some patients (particularly those with very low peak cough flows) cough assist machines can improve lung clearance and reduce hospital admissions due to lower respiratory tract infections.

Availability of early intervention with antibiotics may be critical for some patients with respiratory failure and many will have a supply of antibiotics at home for this purpose. Vaccination against influenza, COVID and pneumococcal infections is also important. Saliva management (using glycopyrronium bromide, amitriptyline, hyoscine or botulinum toxin injections) may also be essential for those with swallowing problems.

Cardiac complications

Cardiac complications occur with a number of muscle conditions (see Table 9.3). These complications are broadly divided into rhythm disturbances and

Table 9.2 Neuromuscular conditions associated with respiratory failure

	Respiratory failure	Rarely respiratory failure
Dystrophies	Duchenne muscular dystrophy	
	Becker muscular dystrophy	
	Myotonic dystrophy*	
	Facioscapulohumeral muscular dystrophy	
	Limb girdle muscular dystrophy* R1(2A), R9 (2I), SGCG, SGCA, SGCB, SGCD(2C-F)	
	Emery–Dreifuss muscular dystrophy	
Congenital	Nemaline myopathy*	
	Myofibrillar myopathy* (e.g., desminopathy)	
Metabolic	Acid maltase deficiency* (Pompe disease)	
	Primary carnitine deficiency*	
	Debrancher enzyme deficiency*	
Mitochondrial	Generalised myopathy	Chronic progressive external ophthalmoplegia
	Leigh's disease	
Endocrine/electrolyte disturbance	Hypo-/hyperkalaemia*	
	Hypo-/hypermagnesemia*	
	Hypophosphataemia*	
	Hyperthyroidism*	
	Barium intoxication*	
Inflammatory	Acute neuropathy: acute inflammatory demyelinating polyneuropathy (Guillain–Barré syndrome)	Polymyositis
		Dermatomyositis
Critical illness	Critical illness neuropathy/myopathy*	
Neuromuscular junction	Myasthenia gravis*	
	Lambert–Eaton myasthenic syndrome*	
	Congenital myasthenic syndromes*	
	Botulism*	

* Respiratory failure may be the first presenting feature.

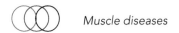

Table 9.3 Neuromuscular disease associated with cardiac complications

	Muscle condition	Cardiac complications
Dystrophies	Duchenne muscular dystrophy	Hypertrophic cardiomyopathy (early), dilated cardiomyopathy (late), arrythmias (atrial and ventricular tachycardia), sudden death
	Becker muscular dystrophy	Arrhythmias, 30% cardiomyopathy, sudden death
	Myotonic dystrophy	Arrhythmias (brady and tachyarrhythmias), progressive heart block, cardiomyopathy uncommon, sudden death
	Emery–Dreifuss muscular dystrophy	Arrhythmias: sinus bradycardia (early), atrial tachycardia, AV conduction block (late), cardiomyopathy, sudden death 50%
	Limb girdle muscular dystrophy D1 (1A) Myofibrillar myopathy Myotilin	Cardiomyopathy, arrhythmias
	Limb girdle muscular dystrophy D2 (1B), laminin AC	Arrhythmias, cardiomyopathy
	Limb girdle muscular dystrophy SGCG, SGCA, SGCB, SGCD(2C-F), sarcoglycanopathies	Cardiomyopathy
	Limb girdle muscular dystrophy R9 (2I), fukutin-related protein (FKRP)	Cardiomyopathy
	X-linked scapuloperoneal muscular dystrophy	Hypertrophic cardiomyopathy
Inflammatory	Primary inflammatory myopathies	Arrhythmias, cardiomyopathy (uncommon), myocarditis
Metabolic	Carnitine deficiency	Cardiomyopathy
	Acid maltase deficiency	Cardiomyopathy
	Debrancher enzyme deficiency	Cardiomyopathy

(Continued)

Table 9.3 (Continued)   Neuromuscular disease associated with cardiac complications

	Muscle condition	Cardiac complications
Mitochondrial	Kearns–Sayre syndrome	Arrhythmias (bradycardia), dilated cardiomyopathy (late), sudden death
Channelopathy	Andersen–Tawil syndrome	Arrhythmias: prolonged QT (early), bidirectional ventricular tachycardia, bigeminy, conduction block (late); valvular abnormalities, sudden death
Neuromuscular junction	Myasthenia gravis	Myocarditis

cardiomyopathy. Rhythm disturbances may be treated by anti-arrhythmic drugs, ablation procedures, pacemakers and implantable defibrillators. Cardiomyopathy is usually treated with β-blockers and ACE inhibitors, but a heart transplant may also be an option.

Routine electrocardiograms and echocardiograms are required in those with conditions associated with these complications. For some patients, for example, those with Emery–Dreifuss muscular dystrophy, the risk of sudden cardiac death is high and these patients require closer monitoring. In some conditions, such as Emery–Dreifuss muscular dystrophy and Duchenne muscular dystrophy, there is an increased risk of cardiac complications in both manifesting and non-manifesting carriers, so family members who are gene carriers should also receive cardiac screening.

Other management

Exercise and rehabilitation programmes may make considerable improvements in function and delay disability. Surgery may be required for kyphoscoliosis, contractures and deformity (e.g., of the feet).

Good nutritional surveillance and intervention, pain management and excellent psychological support are also important determinants of health, quality of life and the ability to live independently at home.

Whilst the frontiers of medical science move forward in developing new treatments, much of the impact that healthcare can make on the quality of life lies in careful consideration of the needs of individual patients. A multidisciplinary team that can accompany a patient on their journey, responding swiftly and flexibly to their needs over time and providing support with compassion and kindness is essential for providing the best care for people living with neuromuscular conditions.

Further reading

Ashizawa T et al. 2019. Consensus-based care recommendations for adults with myotonic dystrophy type 1. *Neurology Clinical Practice* 8(6): 507–520.

Bibekananda K, Santiago CR, Sabharwal A, Clark KJ & Ekker SC. 2023. Mitochondrial base editing: recent advances towards therapeutic opportunities. *Int J Mol Sci* 24(6): 5798.

Birnkrant D et al. 2018. Diagnosis and management of Duchenne muscular dystrophy, part 1: diagnosis and neuromuscular rehabilitation, endocrine, gastrointestinal and nutritional management. *Lancet Neurol* 17(3): 251–267.

Birnkrant D et al. 2018. Diagnosis and management of Duchenne muscular dystrophy, part 2: respiratory, cardiac, bone health and orthopaedic management. *Lancet Neurol* 17(4): 347–361.

Birnkrant D et al. 2018. Diagnosis and management of Duchenne muscular dystrophy, part 3: primary care, emergency management, psychosocial care and transitions of care across the lifespan. *Lancet Neurol* 17(5): 445–455.

Cheng PC, Panitch HB & Hansen-Flaschen JH. 2020. Transition of patients with neuromuscular disease and chronic ventilator-dependent respiratory failure from pediatric to adult pulmonary care. *Paediatr Respir Rev* 33: 3–8.

Dalakas MC. 2023. Autoimmune inflammatory myopathies. *Handbook Clinical Neurology* 195: 425–460.

Hansen-Flaschen J & Ackrivo J. 2023. Practical guide to management of long-term non-invasive ventilation for adults with chronic neuromuscular disease. *Respirat Care* 68(8): 1123–1157.

Magot A, Wahbi K, Leturcq F, Jaffre S, Pereon Y & Sole G. French BMD working group. 2023. Diagnosis and management of Becker muscular dystrophy: the French guidelines. *J Neurol* Jul 9. doi:19.1007/s00415-023-11837-5.

Mercuri E, Finkel RS, Muntoni F, Wirth B, Montes, J, Main M, Mazzone ES, Vitale M, Snyder B, Quijano-Roy S, Bertini E, Hurst Davis R, Meyer OH, Simonds AK, Schroth MK, Graham RJ, Kirschner J, Iannaccone ST, Crawford TO, Woods S, Qian Y & Sejersen T. 2018. Diagnosis and management of spinal muscular atrophy: Part 1: Recommendations for diagnosis, rehabilitation, orthopaedic and nutritional care. *Neuromuscul Disord* 28(2): 103–115.

Mercuri E, Finkel RS, Muntoni F, Wirth B, Montes, J, Main M, Mazzone ES, Vitale M, Snyder B, Quijano-Roy S, Bertini E, Hurst Davis R, Meyer OH, Simonds AK, Schroth MK, Graham RJ, Kirschner J, Iannaccone ST, Crawford TO, Woods S, Qian Y & Sejersen T. 2018. Diagnosis and management of spinal muscular atrophy: Part 2: Pulmonary and acute care; medications, supplements and immunizations; other organ systems and ethics. *Neuromuscul Disord* 28(3): 197–207.

Monda E, Bakalakos A, Rubino M, Verrillo F, Diana G, de Michele G, Altobelli I, Lioncino AP, Falco L, Palmiero G, Elliott PM & Limongelli G. 2023. Targeted therapies in pediatric and adult patients with hypertrophic heart disease: from molecular pathophysiology to personalized medicine. *Circ Heart Failure* Jul 21. 123.010687.

Nishio H, Niba ETE, Saito T, Okamoto K, Takeshima Y & Awano H. 2023. Spinal muscular atrophy: the past, present and future of diagnosis and treatment. *Int J Mol Sci* 24(15): 11939.

Patterson G, Conner H, Groneman M, Blavo C & Parmar MS. 2023. Duchenne muscular dystrophy: current treatment and emerging exon skipping and gene therapy approach. *J Pharmacol* 15(947): 175675.

Roberts TC, Wood MJA & Davies KE. 2023 Therapeutic approaches for Duchenne muscular dystrophy. *Nat Rev Drug Discov* Aug 31. doi:10.1038/s41573-023-00775-6.

Shah MNA & Yokota T. 2023. Cardiac therapies for Duchenne muscular dystrophy. *Ther Adv Neurol Disord* Jul 3 16: 17562864231182934.

Simonds AK. 2016. Home mechanical ventilation: an overview. *Ann Am Thorac Soc* 13(11): 2035–2044.

Stoodley J, Vallejo-Bedia F, Seone-Miraz D, Debasa-Mouce, Wood MJA & Varela MA. 2023. Application of antisense conjugates for the treatment of myotonic dystrophy type 1. *Int J Mol Sci* 24(3): 2697.

Straub V & Guglieri M. 2023. An update on Becker muscular dystrophy. *Curr Opin Neurol* 36(5): 450–454.

Taran S, McCredie VA & Goligher EC. 2022. Non-invasive and invasive mechanical ventilation for neurologic disorders. *Handb Clinical Neurology* 189: 361–386.

Timchenko L. 2022. Development of therapeutic approaches for myotonic dystrophies type 1 and type 2. *Int J Mol Sci* 23(18): 10491.

Toussaint M, Wijkstra PJ, McKim D, Benditt J, Winck JC, Nasilowski J & Borel JC. 2022. Building a home ventilation programme: population, equipment, delivery and cost. *Thorax* 77(11): 1140–1148.

Viscomi C & Zeviani M. 2023. Experimental therapy for mitochondrial diseases. *Handb Clin Neurol* 194: 259–277.

Vivekanandam V, Jayaseelan D & Hanna MG. 2023. *Handb Clin Neurol* 195: 521–532. doi:10.1016/B978-0-323-98818-6.00006-6

CHAPTER 10
CLOSING COMMENTS

Stefen Brady

Most primary myopathies, hereditary and inflammatory, are rare. Despite this, doctors or allied healthcare professionals in medical and surgical specialities, primary care, emergency medicine, psychiatry and anaesthetics will meet patients with an undiagnosed or diagnosed myopathy. As myopathies are often multisystem disorders, a patient's presenting complaint can be something other than limb weakness obscuring the underlying diagnosis. A few of many examples include presenile cataracts in myotonic dystrophy type 1, cardiomyopathy in manifesting carriers of Duchenne muscular dystrophy, respiratory failure and pulmonary fibrosis in antisynthetase syndromes, dysphagia in inclusion body myositis, contractures in collagen VI-related myopathies, and malignant hyperthermia in *RYR1*- and *CACNA1S*-related disease. Our aim in writing this book was to produce an approachable and informative, but not overwhelming, introduction to a fascinating group of patients and diseases that are often overlooked and underserved by medical services. We very much hope that you find this book a useful (and interesting) introduction to the varied world of myopathies.

DOI: 10.1201/9780429429323-10

CASES

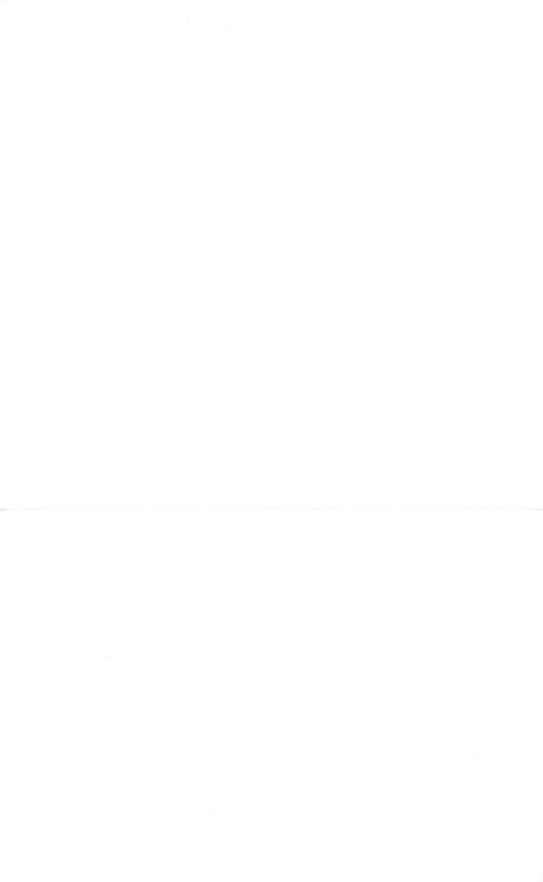

CASE 1

Stefen Brady

PATIENT ASSESSMENT

History

A 22-year-old man was admitted to hospital *in extremis* with shortness of breath at rest and low oxygen saturations (SaO_2 86% on room air). He recounted being unable to climb stairs for several months due to shortness of breath and being unable to lie flat in bed. Initial clinical examination and investigations were consistent with cardiac failure and treatment for this was commenced.

Although his clinical status improved with this treatment, it was subsequently noted once he was better that he could not rise from a seated position without using his arms. Further history revealed lifelong exercise intolerance and poor academic performance out of keeping with that of his sisters. He had no family history of note.

Examination

There was marked wasting of his quadriceps muscles and bilateral Achilles tendon contractures were observed along with bilateral mild–moderate weakness of shoulder abduction (MRC grade 4/5) and hip flexion (3/5) with marked weakness of knee extension (2/5).

Investigations

Serum creatine kinase (CK) level was raised (2538 U/L; normal 40–320 U/L). An echocardiogram revealed dilated cardiomyopathy.

DIAGNOSIS

Becker muscular dystrophy (BMD) due to an in-frame deletion affecting *DMD*.

Discussion

Becker muscular dystrophy (BMD) and Duchenne muscular dystrophy (DMD) are X-linked recessive muscle disorders arising from pathogenic variants in the *DMD* gene encoding the protein dystrophin, which forms an important part of the cytoskeleton of muscle fibres. DMD is the clinically more severe form affecting males in early childhood. In contrast, BMD is less severe sometimes arising later in life. The incidence of DMD is 1:3500–1:6000 live male births. Estimates for BMD vary, but it is approximately one-third as common as DMD. Between 10% and 20% of women carrying a pathogenic variant in *DMD* will develop clinical features. The severity varies widely due to mosaicism. Affected women are called manifesting carriers.

Typical BMD includes calf hypertrophy, combined with limb girdle weakness, and CK levels 5–20 times greater than normal in childhood. However, BMD is phenotypically heterogeneous and other presentations include exercise-induced myalgia and myoglobinuria, prominent quadriceps wasting and X-linked cardiomyopathy. Although onset in childhood is usual, BMD can present at any age including late adulthood (1). Extramuscular features include cognitive impairment (although usually less severe than observed in DMD), psychiatric disorders and cardiomyopathy.

Cardiac disease (cardiomyopathy, conduction block and arrhythmia) is the primary cause of death among patients with BMD. Most affected individuals will develop cardiomyopathy by the third decade of life emphasising the importance of regular cardiac assessment. There is no correlation between the severity of skeletal muscle weakness and the degree of cardiac involvement in patients with BMD and DMD. The optimal management of BMD-related cardiac disease is uncertain. Treatment includes pharmacological therapy such as angiotensin-converting enzyme inhibitors and β-blockers, but when to start such treatment is unknown. Defibrillators and/or pacemaker devices are inserted if clinically warranted. A cardiac transplant may be considered in some cases.

Molecular genetic testing for deletions and duplications in the *DMD* gene is the appropriate initial investigation in boys and men with typical clinical presentations of DMD or BMD. *DMD* is a large gene comprising 79 exons. Eighty per cent of cases of BMD are due to an intragenic deletion. The milder phenotype in BMD relates to the preservation of the genetic reading frame, which results in the production of some dystrophin compared to none in DMD. Although genetic testing has reduced the need for muscle biopsy in cases of DMD and BMD, in atypical presentations or with uncertain genetic results, muscle biopsy can be helpful. Typical findings are dystrophic changes (increased connective tissue, muscle fibre splitting and atrophy, internal nuclei, and muscle fibre necrosis and regeneration) combined with a complete or partial loss of immunohistochemical

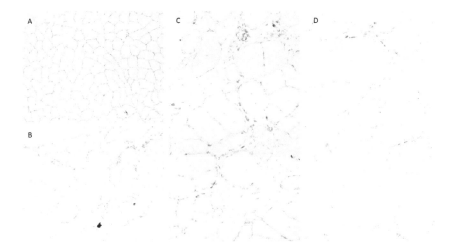

Figure C1.1 Becker muscular dystrophy (BMD). (A) Normal control demonstrating strong positive diffuse sarcolemmal dystrophin immunostaining. Panels B to D show dystrophin immunostaining in BMD. (B) Dystrophin 1 (rod domain) showing relative preservation of sarcolemmal staining. (C) Dystrophin 2 (C terminus) showing reduced but variable sarcolemmal staining in dystrophic muscle. (D) Dystrophin 3 (N terminus) showing patchy loss of sarcolemmal staining.

staining of sarcolemmal dystrophin (see Figure C1.1). Rarely, advanced laboratory techniques such as immunoblotting and mRNA studies are performed.

Learning points

- BMD is associated with several phenotypes including limb girdle weakness, prominent quadriceps wasting and weakness, exercise-induced myalgia and myoglobinuria, and X-linked cardiomyopathy.
- BMD shows a milder clinical phenotype compared to DMD due to the production of some dystrophin protein.
- If the clinical phenotype is indicative of BMD (or DMD), the appropriate initial test is molecular genetic testing for deletions and duplications in the *DMD* gene.
- Despite the presence of two X-chromosomes, 10–20% of female carriers of pathogenic variants in *DMD* will develop symptoms, so-called manifesting carriers. All female carriers should undergo periodic cardiac review.

Further reading

1. Tselikas L, *et al*. Dystrophie musculaire de Becker à révélation tardive. À propos d'un nouveau patient et de 12 observations de la littérature [Late onset Becker muscular dystrophy. A case report and literature review]. Rev Med Interne. 2011;32:181–6.

CASE 2

Sithara Ramdas

PATIENT ASSESSMENT

History

A 4-year-old boy was referred because of a history of frequent falls and difficulty in keeping up physically with his peers. He was mildly delayed in his gross motor milestones, cruising at 14 months and walking independently at 18 months. There were no concerns regarding fine motor skills, language or cognition. There was no family history of note.

Examination

On examination, bilateral calf hypertrophy was observed. He used Gower's manoeuvre when rising to stand. He had weakness of neck flexion (3/5) and hip flexion weakness (2/5) with sub-gravity hip extension. He had no weakness in the knees, ankles and upper limbs. Deep tendon reflexes were elicitable in both the upper and lower limbs.

Investigations

His creatine kinase (CK) level was found to be markedly elevated at 15,000 U/L (normal 40–320 U/L). Genetic testing led to a diagnosis.

DOI: 10.1201/9780429429323-13

DIAGNOSIS

Duchenne muscular dystrophy (DMD) due to an out-of-frame deletions of exons 46–49.

Discussion

Duchenne muscular dystrophy (DMD) is an X-linked recessive disorder arising because of pathogenic variants in *DMD* encoding the large cytoplasmic protein dystrophin, which plays a vital part in muscle contraction. The incidence of DMD is 1:3500–1:6000 live male births.

The typical clinical presentations include boys with gross motor delay or motor difficulties (including frequent falls or difficulty with running and/or climbing stairs), global developmental delay and/or isolated speech delay, as muscle weakness may not be obvious in young infants. In some cases, the only evidence may be an isolated elevated CK level of 20–100× normal. Isolated raised transaminases (aspartate aminotransferase and alanine aminotransferase) in combination with otherwise normal liver function tests should also raise the suspicion of DMD in a boy.

Common comorbidities associated with DMD include learning difficulties (30%), autism spectrum disorder (15%), attention-deficit hyperactivity disorder (32%) and anxiety (27%).

Molecular genetic testing for DMD is the appropriate initial investigation in boys if the diagnosis is suspected. Seventy per cent of boys with DMD have a single-exon or multi-exon deletion, or duplication detected by multiplex ligation-dependent probe amplification (MLPA) or microarray. The remaining 25–30% require next-generation sequencing to detect point mutations (nonsense or missense), small deletions, small duplications or insertions in *DMD*. When performed, muscle biopsy usually reveals dystrophic changes and absent staining for all isoforms of the dystrophin gene (rod, N-terminus and C-terminus), although reduced or patchy dystrophin staining may be observed (Figure C2.1).

Glucocorticoids are the mainstay of current treatment. Benefits include delayed age at loss of ambulation, better preservation of respiratory function and reduction in the requirement for scoliosis surgery. The side effects of long-term glucocorticoid use are not negligible, and active monitoring for reduced growth velocity, pubertal delay, bone demineralisation, weight gain, adrenal suppression, adverse behaviour issues, hypertension, glucose intolerance, cataracts and gastritis, is necessary and important.

Several mutation-specific treatments have regulatory approval including ataluren (nonsense mutations – EMA), eteplirsen (exon 51 skippable mutations – FDA), viltolarsen and golodirsen (exon 53 skippable mutations – FDA), casimersen (exon 45 skippable mutations – FDA). However, these medications are not universally available.

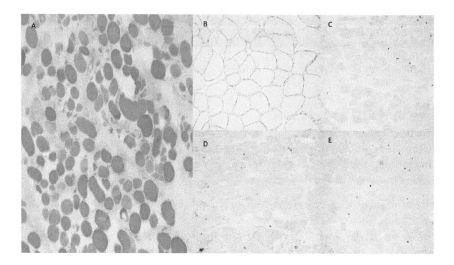

Figure C2.1 Duchenne muscular dystrophy. A. Haematoxylin and eosin (20x) demonstrating dystrophic muscle with moderate variation, scattered necrotic fibres and increased endomysial connective tissue replacing normal muscle. B. Dystrophin control staining demonstrating strong positive diffuse sarcolemmal staining in normal muscle. C. Dystrophin 1 (rod domain) showing complete loss of sarcolemmal staining. D. Dystrophin 2 (C terminus) showing complete loss of sarcolemmal staining. E. Dystrophin 3 (N terminus) showing complete loss of sarcolemmal staining.

Respiratory involvement is universal in DMD and usually progresses following loss of ambulation. An anticipatory approach with regular spirometry, timely initiation of lung volume recruitment, assisted coughing, nocturnally assisted ventilation and subsequent daytime ventilation can improve quality of life and increase survival. Cardiovascular complications are currently the main cause of disease-related morbidity and mortality in those with DMD. Prophylactic use of ACE (angiotensin-converting enzyme) inhibitors by the age of 10 years in asymptomatic boys (without evidence of abnormality on echocardiogram or cardiac MRI) is the current recommended practice.

Two-thirds of mothers of an affected child will carry the *DMD* pathogenic variant. In those, an echocardiogram is recommended every 3–5 years to monitor for the development of a cardiomyopathy. Twenty per cent of female carriers will develop progressive muscle weakness, but usually to a lesser severity than the males. These individuals are termed "manifesting carriers".

Learning points

- DMD is most often associated with progressive limb girdle weakness but may also present with developmental delay in young boys in whom muscle weakness may not be obvious.
- Current treatments delay the progression of the disease but DMD remains a significantly life-limiting condition due to its associated cardiac and respiratory morbidity.

- Genetic testing for DMD should be performed in all boys who present with motor difficulties and raised CK or with a significantly raised CK level in isolation. However, the diagnosis may also be considered in girls with a limb girdle pattern of weakness and accompanying elevated CK levels.
- Two thirds of mothers with an affected child carry the DMD pathogenic variant and will require lifelong cardiac screening.
- Long-term management requires multidisciplinary team input.

Further reading

Birnkrant D et al. Diagnosis and management of Duchenne muscular dystrophy, part 1: diagnosis, and neuromuscular, rehabilitation, endocrine, and gastrointestinal and nutritional management. *Lancet Neurol.* 2018 Mar;17(3):251–267.

Birnkrant D et al. Diagnosis and management of Duchenne muscular dystrophy, part 2: respiratory, cardiac, bone health, and orthopaedic management. *Lancet Neurol.* 2018 Apr;17(4):347–361.

Birnkrant D et al. Diagnosis and management of Duchenne muscular dystrophy, part 3: primary care, emergency management, psychosocial care, and transitions of care across the lifespan. *Lancet Neurol.* 2018 May;17(5):445–455.

CASE 3

Stefen Brady

History

A 58-year-old man was referred to the muscle clinic with a diagnosis of a genetically undetermined distal myopathy. He presented with a 10-year history of progressive bilateral foot drop. Investigations prior to referral included a creatine kinase (CK) level of 556 IU/L (40–320 IU/L), electromyography (EMG) revealing myopathic changes in several lower limb muscles, a muscle biopsy (Figure C3.1) from the tibialis anterior muscle showed variation in fibre size and split fibres, and electron microscopy revealed areas of myofibrillar disorganisation.

Further history elicited from the patient and his partner uncovered that he had never been able to whistle and slept with his eyes partially open. Since his 20s, he had struggled with shoulder pain and had difficulty performing tasks such as changing bed sheets and hanging up washing. More recently, climbing upstairs had become difficult for him. There was no family history of note.

Examination

He had prominent cheekbones and lips consistent with atrophy of the lower facial muscles. Periocular (Bell's phenomenon) and perioral (inability to purse lips and transverse smile) weakness were evident.

Further examination findings were transverse axillary creases and pectoral muscle wasting, asymmetric scapular winding (scapula alata), upper arm wasting with preservation of the deltoid muscles (Figure C3.2), moderate asymmetric weakness of elbow extension (MRC grading 3/5), moderate weakness of hip flexion (3/5) and knee extension (3/5), and marked weakness of ankle dorsiflexion (0/5).

Additional signs were a protuberant abdomen out-of-keeping with his body habitus, positive Beevor's sign (indicative of lower abdominal weakness) and increased lumbar lordosis.

DOI: 10.1201/9780429429323-14

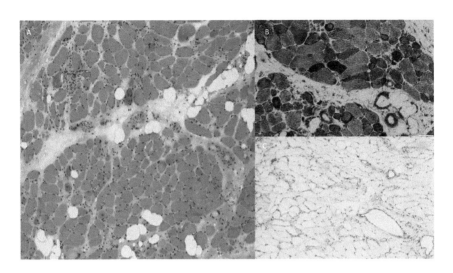

Figure C3.1 (A) Haematoxylin and eosin stain highlights dystrophic muscle with variation in fibre diameters, including numerous hypertrophied fibres, focal necrosis, patchy inflammation (arrow), and increased endomysial connective tissue and interstitial fat. (B) Nicotinamide adenine dinucleotide (NADH) histochemical stain demonstrating abnormal myofibrillar architecture including lobulated and moth-eaten fibres. (C) Immunohistochemical inflammatory marker beta-2 macroglobulin (also known as major histocompatibility complex (MHC) class I) revealing diffuse upregulation of sarcolemmal expression on all muscle fibres.

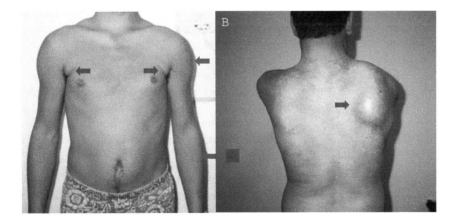

Figure C3.2 Clinical photographs showing (A) transverse axillary creases (blue arrows) indicating atrophy of the pectoral muscles with wasting of the upper arm muscles with preservation deltoid and forearm muscles (red arrows), and (B) marked asymmetric scapular winging (blue arrow).

DIAGNOSIS

Facioscapulohumeral muscular dystrophy (FSHD) due to truncation of D4Z4 repeat sequence on chromosome 4qA.

Discussion

Facioscapulohumeral dystrophy (FSHD) is one of the commonest muscular dystrophies in the United Kingdom (UK). It is an autosomal dominant disorder. However, a positive family history is frequently absent, as one-third of cases are due to *de novo* mutations. Ninety-five per cent of cases of FSHD, so-called FSHD1, are due to deletion of polymorphic repeats on chromosome 4qA. Most individuals with FSHD have signs of the disease by the end of their second decade. The distribution of weakness is pathognomonic. Disease progression is in a cranio-caudal direction.

Facial weakness affects both the periocular and perioral muscles. Symptoms of the former include dry eyes or family members reporting that the patient sleeps with their eyes open. The latter is identifiable by an inability to drink through a straw or whistle. Facial weakness in FSHD is typically bilateral and as a result, often overlooked. Infrequently, there may be no facial weakness. In such cases, a clue to the diagnosis can be prominent cheekbones and lips due to atrophy of the lower facial muscles. Scapular winging often brings individuals to medical attention, but it is also easily and frequently missed if the patient's clothing is not removed and their back is not thoroughly examined. The deltoid muscles are relatively preserved and, therefore, shoulder abduction strength below shoulder height is often normal or only mildly reduced. Individuals with FSHD were described to have "Popeye" arms because, like the fictional 1920s cartoon character Popeye the Sailor Man, of the preservation of forearm muscles in comparison to the wasting and weakness of the humeral muscles. Ankle dorsiflexion weakness is frequent and may precede pelvic girdle and proximal lower limb weakness. Asymmetric weakness is the norm in FSHD. Examination of the torso reveals several characteristic signs including pectoral muscle wasting evidenced by the presence of transverse axillary creases, a prominent abdomen in contrast to the individual's body habitus with a positive Beevor's sign due to lower abdominal muscle weakness, and increased or marked lumbar lordosis.

Despite the early onset of symptoms and signs, late presentations of FSHD are not uncommon. Atypical presentations include absent facial weakness (10–15%) and camptocormia (bent spine). As observed in this case, foot drop can be a prominent feature and may mislead the unwary clinician if other signs are not sought. Other myopathies that may be initially mistaken for a distal myopathy because of the presence of a marked foot drop include myotonic dystrophy type 1 (DM1), inclusion body myositis (IBM) and Becker muscular dystrophy (BMD).

Extramuscular features reported in FSHD include retinal vasculopathy, hearing loss and supraventricular arrhythmia. However, in typical FSHD these are rarely of clinical relevance and routine surveillance is unnecessary. An important feature of significant clinical consequence in FSHD, but one that is difficult to manage adequately, is pain. It usually affects the shoulders and lower back. Although it is indubitably due in part to muscle weakness leading to abnormal movement and joint instability, it is much more prominent in FSHD than in other myopathies and often present in the absence of significant weakness.

In a clinically typical case, the initial diagnostic test for FSHD is molecular genetic testing, looking for a deletion affecting the D4Z4 repeat sequence on chromosome 4qA. Testing for FSHD is complicated and usually performed in specialist laboratories. A deletion is present in 95% of cases of FSHD, more accurately called FSHD1. Of the remaining 5% of cases, most are due to pathogenic variants in *SMCHD1* and are referred to as FSHD2. The genetic basis of FSHD1 and 2 is fascinating and discussed in Chapter 8. For the interested reader, more detailed publications on the topic are included in the "Further reading" list. Muscle biopsy is rarely performed in FSHD due to the highly sensitive and specific clinical presentation. Histopathological features observed in FSHD are varied and rarely helpful. In rare cases, when the clinical features are missed and a muscle biopsy is performed, the presence of inflammatory changes, one of the protean histopathological features reported in FSHD, can lead the clinician to the incorrect diagnosis of an inflammatory myopathy.

Management of individuals with FSHD is primarily supportive and aims to maximise function through exercise and aids. A small number of individuals may benefit from scapular fixation surgery, which should only be performed by an experienced surgeon in collaboration with a specialist neuromuscular clinic.

Learning points
- FSHD is one of the three commonest muscular dystrophies in the UK. The others are myotonic dystrophy type 1 and the dystrophinopathies, Duchenne and Becker muscular dystrophies.
- Signs of FSHD are usually evident before 20 years of age.
- Clinical examination is characteristic and typically includes facial and scapuloperoneal weakness that progress in a craniocaudal direction.
- The initial investigation is molecular genetic testing for FSHD1.

Further reading
Best practice guidelines on genetic diagnostics of facioscapulohumeral muscular dystrophy: Workshop 9th June 2010, LUMC, Leiden, The Netherlands.

Richard J.L.F. Lemmers et al., Digenic inheritance of an SMCHD1 mutation and an FSHD-permissive D4Z4 allele causes facioscapulohumeral muscular dystrophy type 2. *Nature Genetics* 44(12):1370–4.

Case 4

Andria Merrison

PATIENT ASSESSMENT

History
A 48-year-old man first began to notice lower limb weakness following a series of falls whilst playing squash in his early 20s. Over the course of the next decade, he experienced progressive weakness in the lower limbs (in both proximal and distal muscles) with development of contractures. He had been born normally, achieved normal motor milestones as a child and enjoyed sport throughout childhood and early adult life.

At the age of 37, he began to use a wheelchair. Over several years, he had a number of falls that led to lower limb fractures. From the age of 40, he developed progressive proximal weakness in the upper limbs. By the age of 50, he was unable to weight bear and was using an electric wheelchair. Three years later he required non-invasive ventilation at night.

He had a younger brother who was similarly affected.

Examination
All cranial nerves were intact. There was marked symmetrical wasting of the deltoids, subscapularis, biceps, triceps, glutei, quadriceps and distal lower limb muscles without fasciculation. Reflexes were normal; the plantar flexors and all sensory modalities were intact.

Investigations
Creatine kinase (CK) ranged from 4,000 to 8,000 over a period of years. EMG demonstrated widespread myopathic changes. MRI of the lower limbs demonstrated wasting of the glutei, quadriceps, soleus and gastrocnemius, with marked sparing of hip abductors.

Genetic testing revealed a pathogenic variant in the calpain gene.

   DOI: 10.1201/9780429429323-15

DIAGNOSIS

Recessive limb girdle muscular dystrophy R1 (calpainopathy, previously known as LGMD 2A).

Discussion

Limb girdle muscular dystrophy (LGMD) was described by Walton and Natrass in 1954 as a separate group of conditions, characterised by limb girdle weakness with or without the involvement of other muscle groups. From the 1990s onwards, the identification of disease-causing genes and their protein products has led to an understanding of the forms of LGMD and their wide genetic and phenotypic variability. They have been classified on the basis of their mode of inheritance: type 1 autosomal dominant (8 forms) being less common, and type 2 autosomal recessive (28 forms to date) and most frequently occurring. This group now includes conditions with mainly proximal involvement (LGMD2I), those with mainly distal involvement (LGMD2B) and others with both.

In 2017 the second meeting of the European Neuromuscular Centre (ENMC) was held and led to a consensus for updating LGMD nomenclature and classification. The autosomal dominant forms were named D (from 1 to 5) and the recessive forms R (from 1 to 23).

LGMDs have an estimated prevalence of 2/100,000. There are significant differences in presentation in a number of ethnic groups, in part due to founder mutations. LGMD can present at any age, but some forms tend to arise in childhood (1B, 2C–G, 2J).

Other features of LGMD include muscle wasting or hypertrophy, limb contractures or scapular winging. Extraocular, facial and bulbar muscles are usually spared. Respiratory involvement is common in some forms (1B, 2C–F, 2I) and uncommon in others. Similarly, cardiac involvement is more prominent in some forms (1A, 1B, 2I).

LGMD2A (calpainopathy) is the commonest recessive form of LGMD and is due to mutations in the gene (often in one of seven exomes) for the calcium-dependent cytoplasmic protease enzyme calpain-3. It frequently leads to scapular winging, and wasting of the gluteal and both proximal and distal posterior compartment muscles and contractures. Respiratory involvement is less common and is usually mild and slowly progressive.

Creatine kinase is usually raised (>1500). Whilst calpain staining may be abnormal on muscle biopsy (as well as having dystrophic changes), both immunohistochemistry and immunoblot may appear normal. Lobulated fibres may be seen within the muscle (Figure C4.1). Particular patterns of muscle involvement can be identified with magnetic resonance imaging. Genetic testing confirms the diagnosis.

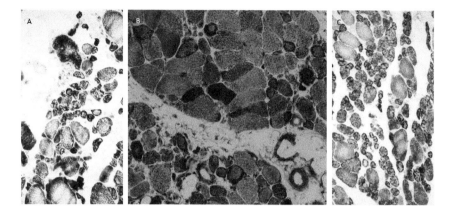

Figure C4.1 Calpainopathy. In addition to non-specific myopathic/dystrophic findings, the presence of lobulated fibres is a common finding in Calpainopathy. These are best observed on the oxidative enzyme stains. A. SDH. B. NADH and C. COX.

Learning points

- Limb girdle muscular dystrophy is an uncommon but important cause of proximal, proximal and distal and rarely distal weakness in both adults and children.
- These conditions are usually recessively inherited, but there is wide genetic and phenotypic variability, even within the same family.
- Diagnosis relies on genetic testing, but clinical examination, CK analysis, muscle MRI and, in some cases, muscle biopsy may be helpful.
- Other causes of proximal weakness should be excluded:
  - With contractures (Emery–Dreifuss muscular dystrophy, Bethlem myopathy, glycolytic metabolic myopathies).
  - With scapular winging (facioscapulohumeral muscular dystrophy, McArdle's disease).
  - With muscle hypertrophy (myotonia congenital, Duchenne/Becker muscular dystrophy).
- A number of forms are associated with respiratory and/or cardiac involvement, and this may be the presenting feature. Lifelong respiratory and cardiac surveillance is required.

References

Bockhorst J & Wicklund M (2020) Limb girdle muscular dystrophies. *Neurologic Clinics* 38(3): 493–504.

Bushby K (2009) Diagnosis and management of the limb girdle muscular dystrophies. *Practical Neurology* 9(6): 314–332.

Lasa-Elgarresta J, Mosqueira-Martin L, Naldaiz-Gastesi N, Saenz A, Lopez de Munain A & Vallejo-Illarramendi A (2019) Calcium mechanisms in limb girdle muscular dystrophy with CAPN3 mutations. *International Journal of Molecular Science* 20(18): 4548.

Norwood FLM, Harling C, Chinnery PF, Eagle M, Bushby K & Straub V (1999) Prevalence of genetic muscle disease in Northern England: in-depth analysis of a muscle clinic population. *Brain* 132: 3175–3186.

Straub V, Murphy A, Udd B & The LGMD Workshop Study Group. (2018) 229th ENMC international workshop: Limb girdle muscular dystrophies – Nomenclature and reformed classification, the Netherlands 17-19 March 2017. *Neuromuscular Disorders* 28(8): 702–710.

CASE 5

Andria Merrison

PATIENT ASSESSMENT

History

A 43-year-old woman presented with a 10-year history of slowly progressive proximal weakness in all four limbs. It was increasingly difficult for her to rise from a seated position, to get out of bed and to carry bags of shopping. She had no previous neuromuscular (or other medical problems) and had represented her school in a number of team sports. She was the youngest of five siblings and had one brother who had been identified to have a raised creatine kinase (CK) following some problems with muscle pain. She had five children who were well.

When this lady first presented to a neurology clinic some years ago, it was thought that she had an inflammatory myopathy – inflammatory indices were initially mildly raised. She was treated with a combination of steroids and other immunosuppressants (including azathioprine, methotrexate and intravenous immunoglobulin). Despite a possible initial improvement in symptoms on initiation of steroids, these treatments had made no difference.

Examination

On examination, there was proximal muscle weakness in all four limbs grade 4–4+/5. There was symmetrical wasting evident proximally in both anterior and proximal compartments in the lower limbs and particular wasting of the supraspinatus and subscapularis in the upper limbs. Other muscle groups were well preserved. There was no facial weakness and the rest of the neurological and medical examination was normal.

Investigations

Her creatine kinase was significantly raised: 14,949 (along with AST 244 and ALP 59) initially and fluctuated over the years from 2,800 to 8,000. A range of other blood tests, including inflammatory indices and dry bloodspot testing for Pompe disease, were subsequently normal. Electromyography showed chronic myopathic changes. An MRI of the muscles showed wasting of the glutei, vastus lateralis, hamstrings, supraspinatus and subscapularis muscles bilaterally. Genetic testing for calpainopathy, dysferlinopathy and fukutin-related protein (FKRP) mutations were negative. Further genetic testing identified the diagnosis.

All immunosuppressants were stopped and she felt better off steroids. She received physiotherapy and made a number of lifestyle changes. She has subsequently been found to have mild respiratory muscle weakness.

   DOI: 10.1201/9780429429323-16

DIAGNOSIS

Recessive limb girdle muscular dystrophy R12 (ANO5 mutation, previously known as LGMD2L).

Discussion

It is important to distinguish between primary inflammatory muscle disease and disorders of muscle with an associated inflammatory component, but this can be very challenging. Systemic manifestations of inflammatory disease, including inflammatory indices, should be looked for. Evidence of inflammation within muscle fibres (particularly non-necrotic fibres), including upregulation of MHC class I proteins (e.g., β-microglobulin) and invasion by inflammatory cells, on the muscle biopsy may be helpful but can be present in both primary and secondary inflammation (Figure C5.1). Failure to respond to immunosuppressants should always make one reconsider a diagnosis of myositis.

Forms of muscular dystrophy which are commonly associated with inflammation and a significantly raised CK include calpainopathy (LGMD2A), dysferlinopathy (LGMD2B) and FKRP-related (LGMD2I) muscular dystrophy. However, this can occur in a number of other more common dystrophies, including dystrophinopathies (DMD, BMD) and sarcoglycanopathies.

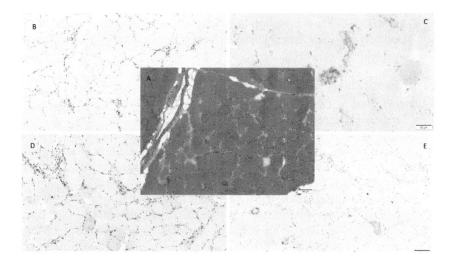

Figure C5.1 ANO5 myopathy. A (centre image) H&E showing non-specific dystrophic findings with fibre size variation, the presence of scattered necrotic fibres, and focal mononuclear inflammation. B. CD68 highlighting myophagia within necrotic fibres. C. Acid Phosphatase highlighting necrotic fibres with myophagia. D. Beta-2-macroglobulin (MHC class II) highlighting upregulation of sarcolemmal expression and occasional necrotic fibres. E. C5b9 (membrane attack complex) showing sarcoplasmic expression in necrotic fibres.

A mutation in the ANO5 gene was first reported to cause a recessive form of limb girdle muscular dystrophy (LGMD2L) in 2010 (Bolduc 2010). This gene encodes for a calcium-channel-activated chloride channel belonging to the anoctamin family of proteins. This channel has been demonstrated to facilitate muscle precursor cell fusion, which is important for muscle repair (Whitlock 2018). A founder mutation was identified in the North and Central Europe population (Hicks 2011) and LGMD2L is now recognised to be the third commonest form of recessive LGMD in this population (Magri 2012, Witting 2013).

Whilst the phenotype is variable, most patients have a relatively mild, slowly progressive form with onset from 20 to 50 years (Hicks 2011, Magri 2012). Cardiac involvement has been reported in some cases (Liewluck 2013). MRI studies (Mahjneh 2012) have shown specific involvement of the gastrocnemius medialis, soleus, hip adductors, hamstrings, gastrocnemius lateralis, quadriceps (and later gluteus minimus and biceps brachialis) muscles. These patients require lifelong cardiac and respiratory surveillance.

Learning points

- Distinguishing primary inflammatory myopathy from secondary inflammation should be considered when symptoms are resistant to immunosuppressants.
- Forms of muscular dystrophy which are commonly associated with inflammation and raised CK are calpainopathy (LGMD2A), dysferlinopathy (LGMD2B), FKRP-related (LGMD2I), dystrophinopathies and sarcoglycanopathies.
- LGMD2L, due to a mutation in ANO5, is the third commonest mutation in North and Central European populations and can also be associated with inflammation.

Further reading

Bolduc V, Marlow G, Boycott KM, Saleki K, Inoue H, Kroon J, Itakura M, Robitaille Y, Parent L, Baas F, Mizuta K, Kamata N, Richard I, Linssen WH, Mahijneh I, de Visser M, Bashir R, Brais B. (2012) Recessive mutations in the putative calcium-activated chloride channel Anoctamin 5 cause proximal LGMD2L and distal MMD3 muscular dystrophies. *American Journal of Human Genetics* 86(2):213–21.

Christiansen J, Guttsches AK, Schara-Schmidt U, Vorgerd M, Heute C, Preusse C, Stenzel W, Roos A. (2022) ANO5-related muscle diseases: from clinics and genetics to pathology and research strategies. *Genes Dis* 9(6):1506–20.

Hicks D, Sarkozy A, Muelas N, Köehler K, Huebner A, Hudson G, Chinnery PF, Barresi R, Eagle M, Polvikoski T, Bailey G, Miller J, Radunovic A, Hughes PJ, Roberts R, Krause S, Walter MC, Laval SH, Straub V, Lochmüller H, Bushby K. (2011) A founder mutation in Anoctamin 5 is a major cause of limb-girdle muscular dystrophy. *Brain* 134(Pt 1):171–82.

Liewluck T, Winder TL, Dimberg EL, Crum BA, Heppelmann CJ, Wang Y, Bergen HR 3rd, Milone M (2013) ANO5-muscular dystrophy: clinical, pathological and molecular findings. *European Journal of Neurology* 10:1383–9.

Magri F, Del Bo R, D'Angelo MG, Sciacco M, Gandossini S, Govoni A, Napoli L, Ciscato P, Fortunato F, Brighina E, Bonato S, Bordoni A, Lucchini V, Corti S, Moggio M, Bresolin N, Comi GP. (2012) Frequency and characterisation of anoctamin 5 mutations in a cohort of Italian limb-girdle muscular dystrophy patients. *Neuromuscular Disorders* 22(11):934–43.

Mahjneh I, Bashir R, Kiuru-Enari S, Linssen W, Lamminen A, Visser MD (2012) Selective pattern of muscle involvement seen in distal muscular dystrophy associated with anoctamin 5 mutations: a follow-up muscle MRI study. *Neuromuscular Disorders* 22 Suppl 2:S130–6.

Soontrapa P & Liewluck T. (2022) Anoctamin 5 (ANO5) muscle disorders: a narrative review. *Genes (Basel)* 13(10):1736.

Whitlock JM, Yu K, Cui YY, Hartzell HC. (2018) Anoctamin 5/TMEM16E facilitates muscle precursor cell fusion. *Journal of General Physiology* 150(11):1498–509.

Witting N, Duno M, Petri H, Krag T, Bundgaard H, Kober L, Vissing J. (2013) Anoctamin 5 muscular dystrophy in Denmark: prevalence, genotypes, phenotypes, cardiac findings, and muscle protein expression. *Journal of Neurology* 260(8):2084–93.

CASE 6

Andria Merrison

History

A 38-year-old woman presented with progressive weakness in all four limbs. She had begun to find it difficult to stand from a seated position, going up and down stairs was more difficult and walking was generally slower. She found it more effortful to wash her hair and to reach up into overhead cupboards in the kitchen.

She had a long-standing history of lipodystrophy dating back to childhood and had always been very self-conscious of her appearance: prominent muscles in her arms and skin changes, including acanthosis nigricans. She reported feeling stiffness in her back since her early teenage years and had not enjoyed sport at school. She developed diabetes mellitus in her 20s.

At the age of 32, she had a series of collapses with associated brief loss of consciousness. A cardiac monitor identified periods of complete heart block and ventricular tachycardia. An implantable defibrillator was used to treat cardiac rhythm problems. She was also receiving treatment for diabetes mellitus.

Examination

Examination of the cranial nerves was normal. There was weakness of shoulder abduction grade 4–/5 despite relatively well-preserved muscle bulk in the shoulder girdle. Similarly, there was symmetrical hip flexion weakness grade 4–/5 without focal wasting or fasciculation. Reflexes were reduced a little and plantars flexor. There were mild contractures of the Achilles tendon bilaterally. Other than a mild reduction in perception of vibration and temperature distally in the lower limbs, sensory function was otherwise normal.

Her skin exhibited multiple skin tags and acanthosis nigricans. She had a wide neck with limited lateral neck flexion.

Investigations

Creatine kinase (CK) was raised at 4884 U/l. Electromyography showed myopathic changes and nerve conduction studies demonstrated a mild axonal neuropathy (attributed to diabetes).

An echocardiogram revealed mildly dilated cardiomyopathy and she was started on lisinopril.

Genetic testing identified a mutation in the laminin A (LMNA) gene. Genetic counselling was provided for family members.

 DOI: 10.1201/9780429429323-17

DIAGNOSIS

Dominant limb girdle muscular dystrophy (laminopathy, Emery–Dreifuss muscular dystrophy 2 EDMD2, previously known as limb girdle muscular dystrophy type 1B).

Discussion

Laminopathy is a rare but increasingly recognised condition with a range of multisystem (skeletal muscle, cardiac muscle, peripheral nerves, fat, bone and skin) phenotypes that usually present in neurological or cardiological practice. The most frequently seen conditions associated with laminin mutations are an autosomal dominant form of Emery–Dreifuss muscular dystrophy (EDMD2, previously known as limb girdle muscular dystrophy type 1B), autosomal recessive Emery–Dreifuss muscular dystrophy and LMNA-related congenital muscular dystrophy.

Laminopathy arises due to mutations in the LMNA gene which encodes for the nuclear envelope proteins laminin A and laminin C. The mechanism of action in determining disease is not fully understood, but disruption of these proteins does appear to disrupt muscle growth (in turn leading to some features such as contractures and a rigid spine). In addition to dystrophic changes (increased fibre size variation, necrotic and regenerating fibres and fibrosis with collagen deposition, and replacement of muscle by fat), fibre type 2 predominance, small type 1 fibres and mild inflammatory changes may be seen on muscle biopsy (Figure C6.1). Specific immunostaining for the laminin A/C proteins is not routinely performed.

Patients present with widely varying degrees of severity of disease. Cardiac involvement shows high penetrance and manifests as conduction defects and dilated (and occasionally restrictive) cardiomyopathy. Most cardiac conduction defects occur before the age of 30 years. Cardiac dysrhythmia and respiratory failure (secondary to respiratory muscle/diaphragmatic weakness) are common causes of death in this group but not all patients have cardiac and/or respiratory muscle involvement.

Most patients with laminopathy have a raised CK. Muscle MRI may identify particular patterns of muscle involvement. Fatty infiltration of the adductor magnus, semimembranosus, long and short heads of biceps femoris and vasti muscles with relative sparing of rectus femoris has been reported.

Identification of a laminopathy does provide an opportunity for genetic testing in other family members. In turn, this can guide cardiac (ECG, cardiac monitoring and echocardiogram) and respiratory screening (lung function tests and overnight oximetry). There is phenotypic overlap with X-linked EDMD, therefore, where appropriate, genetic testing for mutations in emerin may be needed in those who do not have mutations in LMNA. Managing these conditions requires a multidisciplinary approach with good collaboration between neurologists, cardiologists, geneticists and respiratory physicians.

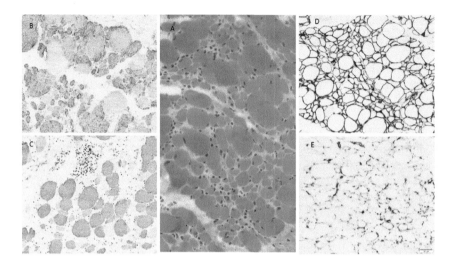

Figure C6.1 Laminopathy (LMNA). A. H&E 10× (central image) demonstrating myopathic changes with clusters of atrophic fibres and hypertrophic fibres with focal inflammation. B. Fast myosin 10× highlighting type 2 fibre predominance and atrophic type 2 fibres. C. Slow myosin 10× highlighting both hypertrophic and a trophic type 1 fibres. Focal inflammation present. D. Laminin alpha 2 immunostains 10× showing preserved sarcolemmal staining and highlights group atrophy. E. Utrophin 10× showing patchy upregulation of sarcolemmal expression.

Learning points

- Laminopathy can lead to multisystem disease and a range of phenotypes, including an autosomal dominant form of muscular dystrophy: Emery–Dreifuss 2 (EDMD2), previously known as limb girdle muscular dystrophy 1B.
- Patients may present in cardiac practice first, and both cardiac (dysrhythmia and cardiomyopathy) and respiratory complications may be life-threatening and require long-term multidisciplinary surveillance.
- There is phenotypic overlap with Emery–Dreifuss muscular dystrophy, so where appropriate genetic testing for mutations in emerin should be conducted in those who do not have mutations in LMNA.

Further reading

D'Ambrosio P, Petillo R, Torella A, Papa A, Palladino A, Orsini C, Ergoli M, Passamano L, Novelli A, Nigro V & Politano L (2019) Cardiac diseases as a predictor warning of hereditary muscle diseases. The case of laminopathies. *Acta Myologica* 38(2): 33–36.

Fan Y, Tan D, Song D, Zhang X, Chang X, Wang Z, Zhang C, Chan S, Wu Q, Wu L, Wang S, Yan H, Ge L, Yang H, Mao B, Bonneman C, Liu J, Wang S, Yuan Y, Wu X, Zhang H & Xiong H (2021) Clinical spectrum and genetic variations of LMNA-related muscular dystrophies in a large cohort of Chinese patients. *Journal of Medical Genetics* 58(5): 326–333.

Lin H, Liu X, Zhang W, Liu J, Zuo Y, Xiao J, Zhu Y, Yuan Y & Wang ZX (2018) Muscle magnetic resonance imaging in patients with various clinical subtypes of LMNA-related muscular dystrophy. *Chinese Medical Journal* 131(12): 1472–1479.

Muchir A, Bonne G, van der Kooi AJ, et al. (2000) Identification of mutations in the gene encoding laminin A/C in autosomal dominant limb girdle muscular dystrophy with atrioventricular conduction disturbances. *Human Molecular Genetics* 9: 1453–1459.

Owens D, Messeant J, Moog S, Viggars M, Ferry A, Mamchaoui K, Lacene E, Romero N, Brull A, Bonne G, Butler-Browne G & Coirault C. (2020) Lamin-related congenital muscular dystrophy alters mechanical signalling and skeletal muscle growth. *International Journal of Molecular Science* 22(1): 306.

CASE 7

Stefen Brady

History

A 33-year-old woman presented with a 30-year history of progressive limb weakness and joint contractures. She was first seen at 4 years of age and diagnosed with Emery–Dreifuss muscular dystrophy because of delayed motor milestones and joint contractures. She underwent surgery for kyphoscoliosis and Achilles tendon contractures in childhood. Her joint contractures had rendered her wheelchair-bound for many years. She had no cardiorespiratory symptoms and had recently undergone a cardiac workup due to a family history of valvular heart disease. She was one of three female siblings. There was no family history of neuromuscular disease or consanguinity.

Examination

Multiple non-pruritic, small red papules, consistent with keratosis pilaris, were observed over her body, most marked over the extensor surfaces of her limbs. Keloid scars were identified at the sites of previous surgical incisions. She had laxity of the distal interphalangeal joints and elbows, and finger flexion contractures, as well as knee and ankle contractures, and prominent calcaneum. She had mild symmetrical weakness (MRC grading 4/5) of shoulder abduction, elbow flexion, finger flexion and moderate weakness of hip flexion (3/5).

Investigations

Her creatine kinase (CK) level was normal: 125 IU/L (20–200 IU/L). Spirometry showed mild restrictive lung disease. A muscle biopsy performed at 4 years of age revealed marked variation in fibre size and increased endomysial connective tissue and fat. Additional immunohistochemical (IHC) staining did not contribute further to her diagnosis but did demonstrate normal IHC staining for emerin.

DOI: 10.1201/9780429429323-18

DIAGNOSIS

Ullrich congenital muscular dystrophy (UCMD) due to heterozygous mutations in *COL6A1*.

Discussion

Contractures are not infrequently observed in many chronic neuromuscular and neurological diseases. However, prominent early onset contractures are indicative of either collagen VI-related myopathies including Ullrich congenital muscular dystrophy (UCMD) and its milder form, Bethlem myopathy (BM), both of which arise secondary to pathogenic variants in three genes that encode the alpha-chain of collagen VI (*COL6A, COL6B* and *COL6C*) or the genetically heterogenous condition Emery–Dreifuss muscular dystrophy (EDMD). The presence of skin abnormalities, joint laxity and cardiac involvement help to differentiate between these two groups.

Clinical features of UCMD are present at birth or soon thereafter and include hypotonia and weakness, proximal joint contractures, and distal joint laxity. Joint contractures may resolve in the first few years of life only to reappear in later years. Other characteristic features include skin and skeletal abnormalities such as keratosis pilaris, hypertrophic or "keloid" scarring, prominent posterior calcaneum, and the presence of kyphoscoliosis. The level of ambulation achieved is variable and some individuals with this condition may never walk. Respiratory failure requiring ventilatory support is a frequent complication of UCMD.

BM can be thought of as a later onset and milder form of UCMD like Becker muscular dystrophy compared to Duchenne muscular dystrophy. Those affected present within the first two decades of life with proximal weakness, distal rather than proximal joint contractures and distal joint laxity. As in UCMD, joint contractures may resolve only to reappear later in life. Similar skin changes are seen in BM and UCMD. Respiratory failure may also occur in BM. In contrast to UCMD, individuals with BM usually remain ambulant.

In both UCMD and BM, the CK level is often normal or only mildly elevated. Muscle biopsy findings are non-specific and can range from mild to markedly myopathic. Immunostaining of muscle tissue for collagen VI can be performed but is inconsistent, and more reliable testing is achieved through culture and staining of skin fibroblasts for collagen VI. Muscle imaging can aid diagnosis as it may reveal peripheral involvement of the vastus muscles with central sparing in both UCMD and BM and an abnormal central signal in the rectus femoris in BM (Figure C7.1). However, in UCMD, the changes can be overshadowed by the presence of significant widespread fatty atrophy of the muscles.

A clinical diagnosis of UCMD and BM is confirmed by molecular genetic testing. As stated, both UCMD and BM result from pathogenic variants in three genes that encode the alpha-chain of collagen VI: *COL6A, COL6B* and *COL6C*. Typically, UCMD is inherited in an autosomal recessive (AR) fashion, while BM

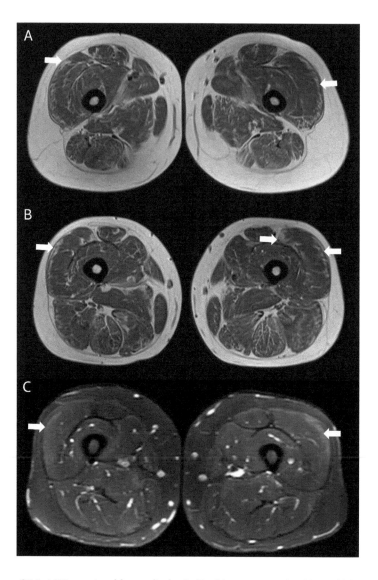

Figure C7.1 MRI proximal lower limbs in Bethlem myopathy. (A and B) T1 axial images through the thigh revealing typical imaging findings in a patient with Bethlem myopathy, peripheral fatty atrophy of vastus lateralis with central sparing (arrows). (C) Earlier in the disease, prior to circumferential fatty atrophy, the same pattern of muscle involvement may be observed on the short-tau inversion recovery (STIR) sequences (arrows).

follows an autosomal dominant (AD) pattern of inheritance. However, cases of AD UCMD and AR BM are described.

The main differential diagnosis for UCMD and BM is EDMD, which is genotypically heterogeneous. Like UCMD and BM, it is characterised by early joint contractures and weakness. However, unlike UCMD and BM, EDMD is associated with cardiac disease including cardiomyopathy, conduction defects and arrhythmias. Further clues to the correct diagnosis are skin abnormalities and joint laxity which are not observed in EDMD. Additionally, muscle biopsy in the commoner X-linked EDMD associated with pathogenic variants in *EMD* demonstrate loss of myonuclear IHC staining for emerin.

Learning points

- Prominent early contractures are observed in collagen VI-related myopathies (UCMD and BM) and EDMD. However, the presence of joint laxity and skin changes in conjunction with the absence of cardiac disease supports a diagnosis of UCMD or BM.
- The clinically more severe UCMD is usually autosomal recessive, while the milder and later onset BM is usually autosomal dominant, though there are rare exceptions to this rule and *de novo* pathogenic variants can occur.
- Muscle imaging and immunohistochemical staining of muscle or cultured skin fibroblasts may aid diagnosis but molecular genetic testing is required to confirm the diagnosis.
- Close monitoring for respiratory failure is necessary.

CASE 8

Andria Merrison

History

A 17-year-old woman presented to a neuromuscular clinic with a clinical diagnosis of congenital myopathy. Her birth and early childhood had been uncomplicated. She had started walking at the age of 2 but was a little unsteady on her feet, and by the age of 5, it was clear that there were problems with mobility. She was found to have significant proximal muscle weakness, initially only in the lower limbs, but this progressed to involve the upper limbs too. By the age of 8 years, she was using a wheelchair and in her teenage life became wheelchair-bound. She had successful surgery for scoliosis at the age of 9.

At the age of 12, her sleep pattern was disrupted and she felt very tired during the day. She was found to have early respiratory failure and non-invasive ventilation was started at night, leading to markedly improved sleep quality and feeling much better during the day. She had had mild swallowing difficulties for 2–3 years.

Examination

On examination, there was bilateral facial weakness, and her tongue movements were slow and speech mildly dysarthric. Neck flexion and extension were weak. There was global muscle wasting, most marked proximally without fasciculation. The tone was normal throughout and there was no evidence of myotonia. There was symmetrical weakness grade 2–3/5 proximally and 4–/5 distally in all four limbs. Reflexes were preserved, and plantar flexors and all sensory modalities were intact.

Investigations

Creatine kinase (CK) and routine blood tests were normal, apart from a low vitamin D level. EMG demonstrated myopathic changes. Muscle biopsy revealed variation in muscle fibre size and multiple rod-shaped structures within myofibres on a number of different histochemical stains (Figure C8.1A–C) but particularly on modified Gömöri trichrome staining (Figure C8.1C). The presence of rods was confirmed with electron microscopy (Figure C8.1D).

Genetic testing subsequently revealed two pathogenic mutations in the NEB gene.

Forced vital capacity was 40% of predicted. Overnight oximetry (without ventilation) showed significant dips in oxygenation overnight.

DOI: 10.1201/9780429429323-19

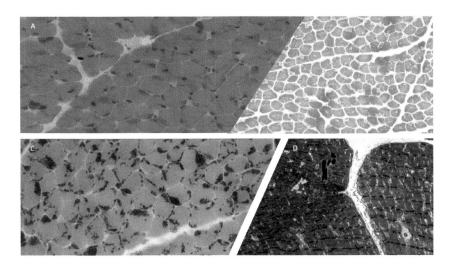

Figure C8.1 Nemaline myopathy. A. H&E 10× demonstrating the presence of many rod-like inclusions within myofibres. B. Metachromatic ATPase 10× showing type 1 predominance ('myopathic' muscle) with absence of staining in areas of rods. C. Modified Gomori Trichrome staining highlighting the presence of numerous 'red' rods in muscle fibres. There are variable numbers present in individual fibres. D. Electron Microscopy confirming the presence of electron dense Z-disk-like material 1–7um in length.

DIAGNOSIS

Nemaline myopathy.

Discussion

Nemaline myopathy is one of the most common forms of congenital myopathy. It is a genetically and phenotypically heterogeneous group of conditions with a wide range of disease severity. Some forms are lethal perinatally or in infancy, others are milder and present in childhood with about 4% presenting in adult life. It usually presents with a slowly progressive form of proximal weakness in childhood, leading to delayed motor milestones. However, patients can present with a late-onset distal myopathy. The more severe intrauterine or perinatal forms may lead to contractures, fractures, absence of movement and/or early respiratory failure.

Mutations in a number of different genes are associated with nemaline myopathy in an autosomal dominant, recessive or sporadic inheritance pattern. These genes all encode proteins associated with the structure or regulation of the thin filament of the skeletal muscle sarcomere. The most commonly causative are mutations in the nebulin (NEB) gene, causing 50% of cases and are mainly recessive. Nebulin is one of the largest known proteins, making the nebulin gene challenging to sequence, and there may be more causative mutations in this gene and it is likely that there are others yet to be identified.

Nebulin mutations are closely followed by mutations in the ACTA1 gene. Less common mutations are found in TPM3 and TPM2, encoding tropomyosin alpha and beta, or myopalladin, all integral structural proteins of the thin filament. TNNT1 and TNNT3 encode proteins of the troponin complex, which is needed for the structure and function of the thin filament during contraction. Other genes reported to cause this condition include KLHL40, KLHL41, CFL2 and LMOD3.

Muscle weakness and wasting are seen in the proximal, facial, neck flexor, tongue and pharyngeal muscles. NEB mutations can cause a distal onset myopathy. Respiratory failure, with diaphragmatic and intercostal muscle weakness, is common and may be the presenting feature. Respiratory surveillance – regular clinical assessment, lung function tests, overnight oximetry and in some cases carbon dioxide levels – is essential for all patients. Scoliosis is a quite common feature. There is rarely cardiac involvement. Ophthalmoplegia is uncommon but has been observed in patients with mutations in KLHL40 or LMOD3, or exceptional cases in NEB.

CK is usually normal or mildly raised. Electromyography often demonstrates myopathic features. Diffuse thigh, soleus and tibialis anterior muscles are commonly seen on MRI in nemaline myopathy. Small case series indicate that ACTA1 demonstrates vasti, sartorius and biceps femoris involvement with relative adductor and gracilis sparing. TPM3 shows involvement in biceps femoris and adductor magnus with relative rectus femoris, adductor longus and gracilis sparing. NEB and ACTA1 both show relative gastrocnemii and tibialis posterior sparing. Increased tiabilis anterior and extensor hallucis longus involvement may correlate with worse mobility.

Nemaline myopathy is characterised by rod-shaped structures (or nemaline bodies) in muscle fibres. These are comprised of thin filamentous material arising from the sarcomere. The subsequent sarcomeric disruption leads to problems with muscle contraction, muscle weakness and wasting. Rod-like structures can also be found in normal myotendinous junctions, normal ocular muscles, ageing muscles and occasionally in other inherited and acquired neuromuscular disorders (including mutations in the ryanodine receptor gene RyR1).

There are currently no curative treatments for nemaline myopathy. Treatments are supportive and aimed at addressing the complications of the condition and improving function and quality of life. Future treatment trials, including gene-modifying therapies, may provide a means of treating people living with nemaline myopathy.

Learning points

- Nemaline myopathy is caused by a range of genes (recessive, dominant and sporadic), most commonly the large nebulin gene, with wide phenotypic variation. These genes all encode proteins associated with the structure or regulation of the thin filament of the skeletal muscle sarcomere.
- Respiratory failure, in particular diaphragmatic weakness, is common in patients with nemaline myopathy and may be the presenting feature.
- The majority of cases are recessive (NEB gene) forms presenting in infancy or childhood, but late-onset (often sporadic) forms do occur and can lead to a rare distal myopathy.

Further reading

Gineste C & Laporte J. 2023. Therapeutic approaches in different congenital myopathies. *Journal Current Opinion Pharmacology* 68: 102328.

Laitila J & Wallgren-Pettersson C. 2021. Recent advances in nemaline myopathy. *Neuromuscular Disorders* 31(10): 955–967.

Naddaf E, Milone NE, Kansagra A, Buadi F, Kourelis R, Naddaf E. 2019. Sporadic late-onset nemaline myopathy: Clinical spectrum, survival and treatment outcomes. *Neurology* 93(3): e298–e305.

Ogasawara M & Nishino IJ. 2023. A review of major causative genes in congenital myopathies. *Human Genetics* 68(3): 215–225.

Perry L, Stimpson G, Singh L, Morrow JM, Shah S, Baranello G, Muntoni F & Sarkozy A. 2023. Muscle magnetic resonance imaging involvement patterns in nemaline myopathies. *Annals of Clinical and Translational Neurology* 10(7): 1219–1229.

Schnitzler LJ, Schreckenbach T, Nadaj-Pakleza A, Stenzel W, Rushing EJ, Van Damme P, Ferbert A, Petri S, Hartmann C, Bornemann A, Meisel A, Petersen JA, Tousseyn T, Thal DR, Reimann J, De Jonghe P, Martin JJ,

Van den Bergh PY, Schulz JB, Weis J & Claeys K. 2017. Sporadic late-onset nemaline myopathy: clinico-pathological characteristics and review of 76 cases. *Orphanet Journal Rare Disease* 12(1): 86.

Younger DS. 2023. Congenital myopathies. *Handbook Clinical Neurology* 195: 533–561.

Yuen M & Ottenheijm CAC. 2020. Nebulin: big protein with big responsibilities. *Journal of Muscle Research Cell Motility* 41(1): 103–124.

CASE 9

Andria Merrison

PATIENT ASSESSMENT

History

A 19-year-old man presented with progressive proximal weakness in all four limbs. He reported that he had not enjoyed sport at school, had been described as a clumsy child and found running very difficult. Getting upstairs had become slow and laboured. He had noticed increasing thinning of his muscles. He described episodes of palpitations.

His maternal grandfather had died suddenly in early adult life, having collapsed due to cardiac complications whilst playing football.

Examination

He had mild facial weakness. There was symmetrical proximal weakness and wasting in all four limbs, most marked in the lower limbs. He had mild contractures in the Achilles and elbow tendons. His heart rate was irregular.

Investigations

Creatine kinase (CK) was 598. ECG showed first-degree heart block and atrial ectopics. The echocardiogram, lung function tests and overnight oximetry were normal. Genetic testing revealed a genetic abnormality in FHL1. A muscle biopsy was not required for diagnosis.

An urgent referral to the cardiology team was made prior to genetic testing.

DOI: 10.1201/9780429429323-20

DIAGNOSIS

Emery–Dreifuss muscular dystrophy.

Discussion

Emery–Dreifuss muscular dystrophy (EDMD) is a rare muscle disease characterised by the clinical triad of progressive muscle weakness, early-onset joint contractures and cardiac involvement. It was first described by British geneticist Alan Emery and German neurologist Fritz Dreifuss in 1966.

EDMD is most commonly an X-linked recessive disorder caused by the gene Xq28, a small gene that codes for emerin. This is a protein localised to the inner nuclear membrane of skeletal and cardiac muscle and present in the cytoplasm of other cells. Some patients have an X-linked dominant form, EDMD1. A variety of mutations have been identified in this gene, causing the absence or reduced expression of emerin. Other pathogenic variants in other responsible genes include LMNA (EDMD2, EDMD3), SYNE1 (EDMD4), SYNE2 (EDMD5) and FHL1 (EDMD6). Congenital forms (EDMD2 and EDMD3) are caused by mutations in laminin A (LMNA), which encodes for A-type laminins, an intermediate filament which has an important role in the cytoskeleton of cardiac and skeletal muscle.

Most patients present with proximal weakness and wasting around 5 years of age, but milder, later onset forms are reported. Patients with FHL1 gene abnormalities can present much later in adult life. Humeroperoneal muscles (often with deltoid sparing) and then later proximal limb girdle muscles are involved. Contractures are seen at the elbows, Achilles and posterior neck tendons. They can become severe with time but need to be actively looked for in early disease. As weakness progresses there is increased lumbar lordosis and a waddling gait. Toe walking, calf hypertrophy and a rigid spine may be present. Scapular winging and mild facial weakness may be seen.

CK may be raised but usually <10× normal. Muscle biopsy, if performed, typically demonstrates dystrophic changes (variation in fibre size, increased interstitial connective tissue, necrotic and regenerating fibres), although the key diagnostic finding is reduced or absent expression of emerin within myonuclei on immunohistochemical staining (Figure C9.1). Skin biopsies are an alternative to muscle biopsy and will show emerin-negative nuclei in both EDMD patients and carriers. More commonly, the diagnosis is confirmed by genetic testing.

EDMD carries a high risk of cardiac complication, including sudden cardiac death (in over 40% of unrecognised cases). Cardiac involvement usually occurs in the second to fifth decade and often leads to atrioventricular conduction block (sinus bradycardia, heart block, atrial flutter and fibrillation). Later in the disease, generalised cardiomyopathy may develop. EDMD is also associated with an increased risk of malignant hyperthermia.

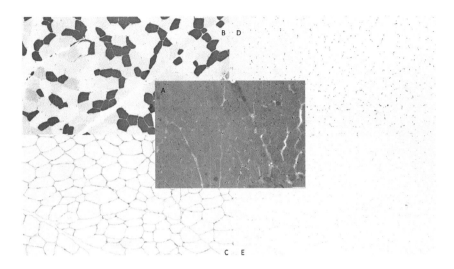

Figure C9.1 Emery Driefuss Muscular Dystrophy. A. H&E 10× showing mild bimodal variation in myofibre diameters. B. Metachromatic ATPase 10× highlighting type 1 smallness. C. Spectrin 10× highlighting the variation in myofibre diameters. D. Emerin IHC 20× `Control' demonstrating retention of nuclear staining in normal muscle. E. Emerin IHC 20× demonstrating widespread loss of nuclear staining confirming the diagnosis of EDMD.

Cardiac monitoring is essential for patients with EDMD and female carriers (who themselves have a 20% risk of cardiac problems). Cardiac pacing and/or implantable defibrillators and medication for cardiac dysrhythmia and/or heart failure may be life-saving. Some patients with progressive cardiomyopathy may be considered for cardiac transplantation.

Learning points

- EDMD carries a high risk of cardiac complications (atrioventricular block and cardiomyopathy) for patients with EDMD and for female carriers, requiring cardiac screening and possible treatment with pacemakers, implantable defibrillators, medication for heart failure and cardiac transplant.
- EDMD is typically associated with significant early contractures (elbows, Achilles, posterior neck).
- Other differential diagnoses for contractures include Bethlem myopathy and calpainopathy (limb girdle muscular dystrophy 2A).
- EDMD is usually X-linked recessive but there are dominant forms (including congenital forms EDMD2).

Further reading

Cannie DE, Syrris P, Protonotarios A, Bakalakos A, Pruny JF, Diaranto R, Martinez-Veira C, Larranaga-Moreira JM, Medo K, Bermudez-Jimenez FJ, Ben Yaou R, Leturq F, Mezcua AR, Marini-Bettolo C, Cabrera E, Reuter C, Limeres Freire J, Rodriguez-Palomares JF, Mestroni L, Taylor MRG,

Parikh VN, Ashley EA, Barriales-Villa R, Jimenez-Jaimez J, Garcia-Pavia P, Charron P, Biagini E, Garcia Pinilla JM, Bourke J, Savvatis K, Wahbi K & Elliott PM. 2023. Emery-Dreifuss muscular dystrophy 1 is associated with high risk of malignant ventricular arryhthmias and end-stage heart failure. *European Heart Journal* 44(48): 5064–5073.

Cesar S, Coll M, Fiol V, Fernandez-Falgueras A, Cruzalegui J, Iglesias A, Moll I, Perez-Serra A, Martinez-Barrios E, Ferrer-Costa C, Del Olmo B, Puigmule M, Alcalde M, Lopez L, Pico F, Berrueco R, Brugada J, Zschaeck I, Natera-de Benito D, Carrera-Garcia L, Expositio-Escudero J, Ortez C, Nascimento A, Brugada R, Sarquella-Brugada G & Campuzano O. 2023. LMNA-related muscular dystrophy: identification of variants in alternative genes and personalized clinical translation. *Frontiers Genetics* 14: 1135438.

De Las Heras JL, Todorow v, Krecinic-Balic L, Hintze S, Czapiewski R, Webb S, Schoser B, Meinke P & Schirmer EC. 2023. Metabolic, fibrotic and splicing pathways are all altered in Emery-Dreifuss muscular dystrophy spectrum patients to differing degrees. *Human Molecular Genetics* 32(6): 1010–1031

Heller S, Shih R, Kalra R & Kang PB. 2020. Emery-Dreifuss muscular dystrophy. *Muscle and Nerve* 61(4): 436–448.

Maggi L, Mavroidis M, Psarras S, Capetanaki Y & Lattanzi G. 2021. Skeletal and cardiac muscle disorders caused by mutations in genes encoding intermediate filament proteins. *International Journal of Molecular Science* 22(8): 4256.

Yunisova G, Ceylaner S, Oflazer P, Deymeer F, Parman YG & Durmus H. 2022. Clinical and genetic characteristics of Emery-Dreifuss muscular dystrophy patients from Turkey: 30 years longitudinal follow-up study. *Neuromuscular Disorders* 32(9): 718–727.

Wang S & Peng D. 2019. Cardiac involvement in Emery-Dreifuss muscular dystrophy and related management strategies. *International Heart Journal* 60(1). 12–18.

CASE 10

Andria Merrison

Andria Merrison

PATIENT ASSESSMENT

History

A 48-year-old woman presented with a longstanding history of progressive distal and proximal muscle weakness affecting all four limbs. At the time of presentation, she was wheelchair-bound.

She recollected developing symmetrical bilateral foot drop during pregnancy at the age of 23 years. She had initially been thought to have a motor neuronopathy. This was followed by progressive proximal muscle weakness in the lower limbs and by the age of 35 years she experienced progressive proximal weakness followed by distal weakness in the upper limbs. She did not report pain, sensory symptoms or sphincter disturbance.

She reported that until recently she had been able to extend her legs (using some remaining quadriceps strength) a little when dangling her legs from a seated position. This had been the last effective movement that she had in her legs.

Examination

On examination, she had no movement in the lower limbs and a flicker of movement in the hands only. She was overweight and muscle definition was difficult to assess. Reflexes were present and symmetrical. All cranial nerves were intact but there was some weakness of neck flexion. Sensory function was normal.

Investigations

Creatine kinase (CK) was 253. Nerve conduction studies were normal but EMG showed widespread severe myopathic changes. A muscle biopsy was attempted but proved technically difficult. Genetic testing for limb girdle muscular dystrophy and myofibrillar myopathies was negative. Further genetic testing established a diagnosis.

DOI: 10.1201/9780429429323-21

DIAGNOSIS

GNE myopathy (hereditary inclusion body myopathy, distal myopathy with rimmed vacuoles, Nonaka distal myopathy).

Discussion

GNE myopathy (previously known as hereditary inclusion body myopathy, Nonaka myopathy, distal myopathy with rimmed vacuoles or quadriceps-sparing myopathy) is a rare autosomal muscle disease characterised by widespread muscle atrophy, which was originally identified in a Japanese population in the early 1980s but is now recognised worldwide. The estimated prevalence is one to nine per million. The gene responsible, on chromosome 9, codes for GNE. Diagnosis depends on identifying pathogenic (homozygous or compound heterozygous, mainly missense) mutations in the GNE gene.

GNE (UDP-N-acetylglucosamine 2-epimerase/N-acetylmannosamine kinase) is an enzyme which catalyses the first two steps in N-acetylneuraminic acid or sialic acid biosynthesis. Modification of glycoproteins and glycolipids (expressed at the cell surface) by sialic acid is crucial for their function in many cell processes, including cell adhesion and signal transduction, and this failure may lead to myopathy. The precise pathological mechanisms for GNE myopathy are not fully elucidated but impaired autophagy may be part of this process.

Symptoms usually begin in the late second or third decade but later onset cases (up to the seventh decade) have been reported and similarly a few cases in children as young as 10 years. Bilateral foot drop, caused by weakness in the tibialis anterior, is the commonest first presentation. Weakness progresses mainly symmetrically in all four limbs, with relative sparing of the quadriceps muscles until later in the course of the disease. Loss of ambulation usually occurs within 10–15 years of onset. The deep finger flexors and intrinsic muscles of the hands are often affected early too.

Cranial nerves are not affected but neck flexion weakness is common. Cardiomyopathy is not associated with GNE myopathy but cardiac dysrhythmia and respiratory muscle weakness are reported infrequently. Thrombocytopenia has been identified in some East Asian families with GNE myopathy.

Serum CK may be moderately raised and EMG is usually myopathic with small motor unit potentials and fibrillation potentials. Muscle MRI may identify early involvement of the biceps femoris short head in some cases.

Muscle biopsy may reveal similar features to inclusion body myositis (hence the previous name) including myopathic changes (type 1 fibre predominance, fibre size variation and variable atrophy) combined with the presence of rimmed vacuoles containing ubiquitinated material. There is increased acid phosphatase activity and lysosomal markers within the vacuoles, suggesting a role for autophagy. In contrast to inclusion body myositis, there is paucity of inflammation and an absence of expression of MHC1 (major histocompatibility complex 1).

Electron microscopy may show filamentous inclusions in the nucleus and cytoplasm, as well as the autophagic vacuoles. Mitochondrial dysfunction, increased amyloid β peptide and reduced sialic acid (important for platelet function) levels have also been found in GNE myopathy.

Although there are no current disease-modifying therapies available, research is underway to develop treatments. Substrate replacement (including increasing sialic acid levels), immunotherapy and gene therapy strategies are being evaluated.

Learning points

- GNE myopathy (hereditary inclusion body myopathy) is a rare condition but should be considered in the differential diagnosis in patients presenting with progressive muscle atrophy, particularly in early adulthood with early bilateral footdrop and late quadriceps sparing (some preservation of hip flexion).
- Other conditions which may feature in the differential for GNE myopathy include the much more common sporadic inclusion body myositis and adult-onset dominant distal and myofibrillar myopathies.
- Cardiac dysrhythmia and respiratory muscle weakness (requiring ventilatory support) may be complications of this condition.
- Diagnosis depends on genetic confirmation and future treatment options may include substrate replacement (sialic acid) and/or genetic modifying therapy.

Further reading

Carrillo N, Malicdan MC & Huizing M. 2018. GNE myopathy: etiology, diagnosis and therapeutic challenges. *Neurotherapeutics* 15(4): 900–914.

Mullen J, Alrasheed K & Mozaffar T. 2022. GNE myopathy: history, etiology and treatment trials. *Frontiers Neurology* 13: 1002310.

Nishino I, Carillo-Carrasco N & Argov Z. 2015. GNE myopathy: current update and future therapy. *Journal of Neurology, Neurosurgery and Psychiatry* 86(4): 385–392.

Nonaka I, Noguchi S & Nishino I. 2005. Distal myopathy with rimmed vacuoles and hereditary inclusion body myopathy. *Current Neurological Neuroscience Reports* 5(1): 61–65.

Pogoryelova O, Gonzalez Coraspe JA, Nikolenko N, Lochmuller H & Roos A. 2018. GNE myopathy: from clinics and genetics to pathology and research strategies. *Orphanet Journal of Rare Diseases* 13(1): 70.

Yoshioka W, Nishino I & Noguchi S. 2022. Recent advances in establishing a cure for GNE myopathy. *Current Opinion Neurology* 35(5): 629–636.

Zhang T, Shang R & Miao J. 2022. The role of amyloid β in the pathological mechanism of GNE myopathy. *Journal Neurological Science* 43(11): 6309–6321.

Case 11

Sithara Ramdas

History

A 6-year-old girl was referred with a history of gross motor delay and ongoing difficulties with gait. She was born at term without any antenatal concerns. She was noted to be floppy and was on nasogastric feeds for 2 weeks. She had recurrent chest infections until 2 years of age. Her gross motor development was significantly delayed. She sat independently at the age of 18 months, stood unaided at 28 months and walked independently at 36 months. But at the age of 6 years, she is unable to run, jump or hop. She required speech and language therapy input for phonation difficulties related to poor lip closure. There are no concerns about her fine motor and cognitive abilities.

Examination

Rise to stand with Gower's manoeuvre. Neck flexion MRC grade 3. Hip girdle weakness was noted with sub-gravity hip extension. Knee extension 4, ankle dorsi flexion 5. Shoulder abduction 4, elbow extension 5, wrist extension 5. Deep tendon reflexes were elicitable in the upper and lower limbs. Mild bilateral facial weakness but the rest of the cranial nerve and cerebellar examination were normal. No spinal rigidity or scoliosis.

Investigations

Creatine kinase (CK) 130 U/L (40–320 U/L).

Muscle biopsy revealed myopathy with cores. Genetic testing established the diagnosis.

 DOI: 10.1201/9780429429323-22

DIAGNOSIS

Congenital myopathy due to compound heterozygous pathogenic variants in *RYR1*.

Discussion

Congenital myopathies are a group of genetic muscle disorders typically characterised by childhood onset of slowly or non-progressive skeletal muscle weakness. Mutations in the skeletal muscle ryanodine receptor (*RYR1*) gene are known to cause both autosomal dominant and recessive muscle disorders. *RYR1* encodes for the sarcoplasmic reticulum calcium release channel (RyR1) which plays a crucial role in excitation/contraction coupling.

RYR1-related myopathy subtypes as based on histopathological features include central core disease (CCD), multiminicore disease (MmD), centronuclear myopathy (CNM), congenital fibre-type disproportion (CFTD) and core-rod myopathy (CRM) (Table C11.1). Other RYR1-related clinical phenotypes now recognised include King–Denborough syndrome, *RYR1* rhabdomyolysis-myalgia syndrome, atypical periodic paralysis, congenital neuromuscular disease with uniform type 1 fibres and late-onset axial myopathy.

RYR1-related myopathy presents with a variable spectrum of clinical features which include early-onset hypotonia, proximal/distal or generalised muscle weakness, facial weakness, ptosis, ophthalmoplegia, bulbar weakness, respiratory involvement (recurrent chest infection, respiratory failure) and orthopaedic conditions (joint contractures, hip dislocation, scoliosis).

All RYR1-related myopathy cases should be considered potentially malignant hyperthemia susceptible; the higher risk is in dominant phenotypes.

Serum CK is normal or mildly raised. Muscle MRI demonstrates relative sparing of rectus femoris and gracilis in CCD-dominant patients with more generalised involvement in other cases.

There are no approved therapies for RYR1-related myopathy. Small studies and case reports have reported benefits with salbutamol and CNM-associated RYR1 myopathy benefits from pyridostigmine. Clinical care due to the multisystem involvement should be via a multidisciplinary team.

Learning points

- RYR1-related congenital myopathy presents with variable age of onset, clinical features, and both dominant and recessive modes of inheritance.
- The main diagnostic investigations in these cases include muscle biopsy and genetic testing. Muscle MRI can aid in diagnosis.
- In most patients, the muscle weakness is stable and non-progressive.
- The risk of malignant hyperthermia should be considered in all patients with pathogenic variants in *RYR1*.
- There are no approved treatments and long-term management requires a multidisciplinary approach.

Table C11.1 RYR1 subtypes and common clinical features

	Hypotonia	Gross motor delay	Weakness	Orthopaedic	EOM weakness	Respiratory	Bulbar
CCD (dominant)	+	+	P, A	+	–	–	–
CCD (recessive)	+	+	G	+	+/–	+	+
MmD	+	+	P, A, D	+	+	+	+
CNM	+	+	P, A D	+	+	+/–	+/–
CFTD	+	+	P, A	+	+	+	+
CRM	+	+	G, A	+	–	+	–

Abbreviations: P, proximal; A, axial; G, generalised; D, distal.

Further reading

Lawal TA, Todd JJ, Meilleur KG. Ryanodine receptor 1-related myopathies: Diagnostic and therapeutic approaches. *Neurotherapeutics*. 2018 Oct; 15(4):885–899.

Wang CH, et al. Consensus Statement on Standard of Care for Congenital Myopathies. *Journal of Child Neurology*. 2012 Mar; 27(3):363–382.

Zhou H, Jungbluth H, Sewry CA, et al. Molecular mechanisms and phenotypic variation in RYR1-related congenital myopathies. *Brain: A Journal of Neurology*. 2007; 130(8):2024–2036.

CASE 12

Andria Merrison

History

A 53-year-old man presented with shortness of breath on minimal exercise and an overall reduction in exercise tolerance soon after a viral illness. He was investigated by the medical team and found to have dilated cardiomyopathy. He was treated for cardiac failure and subsequent problems with cardiac dysrhythmia led to the insertion of a pacemaker and subsequently an implantable defibrillator.

Within a year of his original presentation with cardiac problems, this man began to find it difficult to rise from a seated position and had further problems with being able to sustain exercise. He also reported sleep disruption, unrefreshing sleep and fatigue.

There was a long-standing history of diabetes and mild hypertension. He was also an ex-smoker.

There was a family history of cardiac disease with four family members experiencing premature death (presumed myocardial infarction): his mother at the age of 60, one brother at the age of 60 and one brother at the age of 47, and a maternal aunt at the age of 50 years.

Examination

All cranial nerves were intact. There was weakness of hip flexion grade 3/5 bilaterally and of knee flexion and extension grade 4+/5 bilaterally. Tone was normal throughout and reflexes were present and symmetrical with flexor plantars. There was some wasting of the quadriceps muscles bilaterally without fasciculation. Mild Achilles tendon contractures were evident. Sensory function was normal.

Investigations

Creatine kinase was 8923. Nerve conduction studies were normal, and EMG showed myopathic changes. Echocardiogram revealed dilated cardiomyopathy, lung function tests identified respiratory muscle weakness and overnight oximetry showed nocturnal hypoventilation. A cardiomyopathy gene panel was undertaken, which confirmed the diagnosis.

Treatment

This man received medical treatment for heart failure and was established on nocturnal non-invasive ventilation to improve symptoms of hypoventilation.

 DOI: 10.1201/9780429429323-23

DIAGNOSIS

Myofibrillar myopathy secondary to a BAG3 mutation.

Discussion

BAG3 myopathy is one of the myofibrillar myopathies, a heterogeneous group of neuromuscular disorders characterised by disintegration of the Z-disk, causing disintegration of myofibrils. The BAG3 gene (Bcl-2–associated athanogene 3) encodes a multidomain protein that plays an important role in a number of cellular processes. BAG3 mutations have been reported in a relatively small number of patients. In children, this largely autosomal dominant myofibrillar myopathy leads to rapidly progressive weakness and a poor prognosis with respect to cardiac and respiratory involvement. (De novo mutations have been reported too.) However, in adults, progression may be much slower. Proximal weakness, rigid spine and Achilles tendon contractures are often present.

Muscle biopsy may identify a range of myopathic features including fibre size variability, fibre splitting, excess internal nuclei, increased connective/adipose tissue and/or vacuoles (Figure C12.1). Desmin or myotilin protein accumulation is often observed within affected myofibres. Electron microscopy will highlight myofibrillar disintegration and protein aggregation (Figure C12.2). In addition,

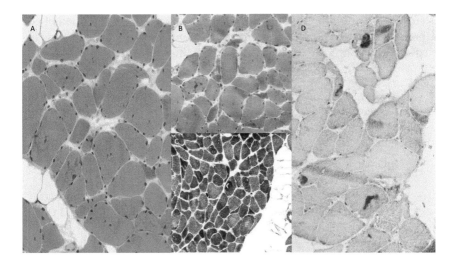

Figure C12.1 Myofibrillar Myopathy. A H&E 10× demonstrating moderate variation in myofibre diameters with split fibres, isolated necrotic fibres and an occasional fibre showing granular eosinophilic material within the cytoplasm. B. Modified Gomori Trichrome 10× highlighting darkly staining material within myofibres. C. NADH 10× confirming many fibres with abnormal/distorted myofibrillar architecture. D. Myotilin immunostains 20× highlighting the presence of abnormal myotilin-positive myofibrillar material within myofibres. A similar pattern of staining was observed for desmin.

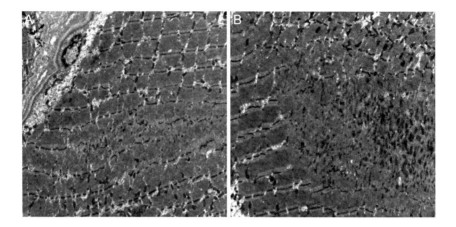

Figure C12.2 Myofibrillar Myopathy. Electron Microscopy images. A. EM of muscle demonstrating disruption of Z-lines. B EM demonstrating accumulation of myofibrillar material.

neuropathic changes may be seen in some BAG3-related cases due to associated polyneuropathy.

BAG is a co-chaperone for heat shock protein HSP70, together contributing to targeting aggregation-prone proteins to macro-autophagic degradation and contributing more widely to anti-apoptosis in a range of degenerative diseases. There is already evidence from in vivo models that transcriptional adaptation of gene expression can prevent myopathy and heart failure, providing encouraging first steps in developing gene-modifying therapy in this condition.

Learning points

- BAG3-related myofibrillar myopathy is rare. Although previously thought of as an autosomal dominant, rapidly progressive condition in children, a wider range of phenotypes, including milder forms presenting in adulthood, are increasingly recognised.
- Proximal muscle weakness, rigid spine and Achilles tendon contractures are common features.
- A number of muscle conditions, including myofibrillar myopathy, may present with cardiac dysfunction as the primary symptom. BAG3 usually leads to cardiomyopathy.
- Gene panels for cardiomyopathy may identify conditions with an associated skeletal myopathy, which may or may not have been evident for the patient prior to testing.
- Respiratory muscle weakness can also be associated with BAG3 mutations.

Further reading

Akaba Y, Takeguchi R, Tanaka R, Makita Y, Kimura T, Yanagi K, Kaname T, Nishino I & Takahashi S. (2022) Wide spectrum of cardiac phenotype in myofibrillar myopathy associated with Bcl-2-associated athanogene 3 mutation: a case report and literature review. *Journal Clinical Neuromuscular Disease* 24(1): 49–54.

Batonnet-Pichon S, Behin A, Cabet E, Dalort F, Vicart P & Lilienbaum A (2017) Myofibrillar myopathies: New perspectives from animal models to therapeutic approaches. *Journal of Neuromuscular Disorders* 4(1): 1–15.

Behin A, Salort-Campana E, Wahbi K, Richard P, Carlier RY, Laforet P, Stojkovic T, Masisonobe T, Verschueren A, Franques J, Attarian S, Maues de Paula A, Figarell-Branger D, Becane HM, Nelson I, Duboc D, Bonne G, Vicart P, Udd B, Romero N, Pouget J, Eymared B & Behin A (2015) Myofibrillar myopathies: State of the art, present and future challenges. *Reviews Neurology (Paris)* 171(10): 715–729.

Diofano F, Weinmann K, Schneider I, Thiessen KD, Rottbauer W & Just S (2020) Genetic compensation prevents myopathy and heart failure in an in vivo model of BAG3 deficiency. *PLoS Genetics* 16(11): e1009088.

Selcen D, Muntoni F, Burton BK, Pegoraro E, Sewry C, Bite AV & Engel AG (2009) Mutation in BAG3 causes severe dominant childhood muscular dystrophy. *Annals of Neurology* 65: 83–89.

Liu L, Sun K, Zhang X, Tang Y & Danyan X (2021) Advances in the role and mechanism of BAG3 in dilated cardiomyopathy. *Heart Failure Reviews* 26(1): 183–194.

Sturner E & Behl C (2017) The role of the multi-functional BAG3 protein in cellular protein control and in disease. *Frontiers in Molecular Neuroscience* 10: 177.

CASE 13

Louisa Kent and Stefen Brady

PATIENT ASSESSMENT

History

A 28-year-old man was seen in the muscle clinic with a 3-year history of progressive difficulty walking. He frequently tripped over his feet and reported falling on several occasions. He found it difficult to grip heavy objects, for example, he experienced difficulty carrying shopping bags. He had no known family history and was otherwise well.

Examination

Examination revealed marked distal lower limb wasting and inability to stand on his heels. Extensor digitorum brevis (EDB) was preserved and he did not have a hanging hallux. There was mild proximal lower limb weakness, with notable sparing of quadriceps. In the upper limbs, there was atrophy of the thenar muscles and weakness of finger flexors. Reflexes and sensation were normal.

Investigations

Creatine kinase (CK) was 1021 IU/L.

Nerve conduction studies were normal. EMG revealed myopathic changes in the distal muscles of the upper and lower limbs.

MRI scan of the legs revealed fatty infiltration in the anterior lower leg muscles bilaterally (particularly anterior tibial and toe extensors) and medial gastrocnemius. In the thighs, there was fatty infiltration of the hamstring muscles but with sparing of the quadriceps.

Muscle biopsy of the left deltoid showed variability in fibre size with many slightly atrophic and angular fibres and some hypertrophic fibres. There was fibre type disproportion with type 1 fibres smaller and more numerous than type 2.

Genetic testing established the diagnosis.

   DOI: 10.1201/9780429429323-24

DIAGNOSIS

GNE myopathy (Nonaka distal myopathy) due to compound heterozygous pathogenic variants detected in *GNE*.

Discussion

The term "distal myopathy" describes a heterogeneous group of slowly progressive inherited myopathies which predominantly affect the distal muscles of either the lower limbs (more commonly) and/or the upper limbs. The classification of distal myopathies is complicated because of the use of eponymous names and varied classification systems that have developed over the years. Previous schemes involving histopathological classification, phenotypic classification and genetic variants have been used. Some distal myopathies are also included in the limb girdle muscular dystrophy (LGMD) classification. In the era of genetics, distal myopathies should preferably be classified (or referred to) by the causative gene. This is not only clearer but provides information on disease course and likelihood of other organ involvement, and can aid in genetic counselling and subsequent family planning.

When presented with a patient with a distal myopathy, careful clinical assessment (history and examination) and investigations (CK, neurophysiology, MRI and muscle biopsy findings) help to narrow the possible causative genes (Table C13.1). The main differential diagnosis for a distal myopathy is distal motor neuropathy. Clinical pointers to the diagnosis of a distal myopathy include distal lower limb weakness with preservation of quadricep strength, retained reflexes and preservation of muscle bulk (particularly of the extensor digitorum brevis). Investigations can further help to distinguish between a myopathy and neuropathy. More often than not the CK will be normal or mildly raised in both distal neuropathy and myopathy. However, CK levels >2000 U/L are almost never neurogenic and point to pathogenic variants of *ANO5* or *DYSF*. Many would consider neurophysiology to be the gold standard for distinguishing a distal myopathy from a motor neuropathy, but it can on occasion be unhelpful especially early in the disease course. Subclinical selective muscle involvement on muscle MRI is sometimes also useful, e.g., in *TTN*-related myopathy there is selective involvement of the anterior compartment in the distal lower limbs, but often it may not add much beyond that which is elicited by thorough clinical examination. A role for muscle biopsy remains, particularly if the phenotype is unusual or a variant(s) of uncertain significance is identified on genetic testing. While no general histopathological features of a distal myopathy exist, some features, such as rimmed vacuoles or myofibrillar aggregates, may point towards certain subsets of distal myopathies.

GNE myopathy is an autosomal recessive distal myopathy which typically presents in early adulthood. It is more prevalent in those of Iranian Jewish descent due to the presence of the founder mutation c.2228T>C (p.M743T) in the population. There is no association with cardiomyopathy, and respiratory muscle weakness is unusual. The most commonly affected muscles initially are the ankle dorsiflexors and toe extensors, often with weakness of finger flexors. This can

Table C13.1 Clinical and muscle biopsy features of rare distal myopathies

Gene	Name(s)	Inheritance	Histopathology	Age at onset	Typical initial distribution of weakness	Other features
TTN	Udd myopathy	AD >AR	Dystrophic with RV	Adult	Anterior lower leg	CM, RF
TIA1	Welander myopathy	AD	Dystrophic with RV	Adult	Hands, finger extensors	
MATRN3	Vocal cord and pharyngeal distal myopathy	AD	Dystrophic with RV	Adult	Distal limb, vocal cord	RF
ACTN2	Distal actinopathy	AD	Myopathic with RV	Adult	Anterior lower leg	CM
NOTCH2NLC, LRP12 and *GIPC1*	Oculopharyngodistal myopathy	AD/AR	RV	Adult	Distal limb, facial, ptosis, bulbar	RF
VCP	VCP-mutated distal myopathy	AD	RV	Adult	Anterior lower leg	Frontotemporal dementia, Paget's disease, ALS
FLNC	Distal ABD-filaminopathy/ C-terminal nonsense mutated distal filaminopathy	AD	Myofibrillar	Early adulthood	Distal lower/ upper limb	CM
DNAJB6	DNAJB6 distal myopathy	AD	Dystrophic with RV	Early adulthood	Distal lower limb	No
MYH7	Laing distal myopathy	AD > AR	Myopathic	Childhood	Anterior lower leg	Hanging toe, CM

(Continued)

Table C13.1 (Continued) Clinical and muscle biopsy features of rare distal myopathies

Gene	Name(s)	Inheritance	Histopathology	Age at onset	Typical initial distribution of weakness	Other features
MYOT	Distal myopathy with myotilin defect	AD	MFM	Adult	Distal lower limb	CM
ZASP	Markesbery–Griggs myopathy Zaspopathy	AD	MFM	Adult	Distal lower limb	CM
DES	Desminopathy	AD >AR	MFM	Adult	Distal lower limb	CM, RF
αB-crystallin	αB-crystallinopathy	AD	MFM	Adult	Anterior lower leg	CM, RF, cataracts
BAG3	BAG3 myofibrillar myopathy	AD	MFM	Childhood	Limb and axial	Neuropathy, CM, RF, rigid spine
PLIN4	PLIN4-associated myopathy	AD	Ubiquitin/p62 positive deposits, RV	Early adulthood	Anterior lower leg	RF
HSPB8	Rimmed vacuolar neuromyopathy	AD	RV	Early adulthood	Anterior lower leg	Neuropathy, RF
KLHL9	Early onset distal myopathy with KLHL9 mutations	AD	Myopathic	Childhood	Anterior lower leg	
CAV3	Distal myopathy with caveolin defect	AD	Myopathic, reduced caveolin3 staining	Early adulthood	Small muscles of hands and feet	Wide phenotype, including LGMD, high CK, rippling muscles

(Continued)

Table C13.1 (Continued) Clinical and muscle biopsy features of rare distal myopathies

Gene	Name(s)	Inheritance	Histopathology	Age at onset	Typical initial distribution of weakness	Other features
DMN2	DNM2-related distal myopathy	AD	Centronuclear myopathy	Childhood/early adulthood	Distal limbs	Ptosis, ophthalmoplegia, facial weakness, RF
RYR1	RYR1 mutated calf predominant distal myopathy	AD/AR	May see core-like structures	Adulthood	Lower/upper limb	Wide phenotype, including rigid spine, malignant hyperthermia
GNE	Nonaka myopathy Distal myopathy with rimmed vacuoles	AR	Myopathic, RV	Early adulthood	Anterior lower leg, hands, sparing quadriceps	
DYSF	Miyoshi myopathy	AR	Myopathic, absent dysferlin staining	Early adulthood	Posterior lower leg, hamstring	Markedly raised CK
ANO5	ANO5 distal muscular dystrophy/distal anoctaminopathy	AR	Scattered necrotic muscle fibres	Early adulthood	Posterior lower leg	Markedly raised CK
NEB	Early onset distal myopathies with nebulin defect	AR > AD	Grouped muscle fibre atrophy	Childhood	Anterior lower leg	
ADSSL	Early onset ADSSL distal myopathy	AR	RV	Adolescent	Weakness in legs > arms	Facial muscle involvement

Abbreviations: AD, autosomal dominant; AR, autosomal recessive; RV, rimmed vacuoles; CM, cardiomyopathy; RF, respiratory failure; MFM, myofibrillar myopathy.

progress to involve more proximal muscles, though quadriceps are often strikingly spared. CK is typically mild-moderately elevated. Muscle biopsy can reveal rimmed vacuoles, perhaps absent in this case due to the choice of a proximal muscle biopsy site.

Learning points

- Distal myopathies are a heterogeneous group of rare inherited myopathies, which in most but not all cases predominantly affect the distal lower limb muscles.
- They are most clearly classified by the genetic cause. Even though some cases still evade diagnosis, detailed clinical assessment will enable the clinician to narrow the differential diagnosis substantially.
- It is important to remember that myopathies such as myotonic dystrophy type 1, facioscapulohumeral muscular dystrophy (FSHD) and inclusion body myositis (IBM) are much commoner causes of distal weakness and should always be considered first.

Further reading

Savarese M et al, Panorama of the distal myopathies, *Acta Myol* 2020 Dec 1;39(4):245–265. doi: 10.36185/2532-1900-028.

CASE 14

Andria Merrison

PATIENT ASSESSMENT

History

A 39-year-old woman presented with a 12-month history of progressive proximal weakness in the lower limbs, longstanding ptosis and mild swallowing difficulties. Her father had experienced progressive proximal weakness in later adult life and now at the age of 71 years was using a wheelchair most of the time. He had undergone successful eyelid elevation surgery and was awaiting a gastrostomy due to worsening dysphagia with associated recurrent chest infections.

Examination

This woman had bilateral symmetrical ptosis, which did not show signs of exacerbation with fatigue. There was some restriction of horizontal and vertical eye movements. She had moderate proximal weakness in all four limbs.

Investigations

Anti-acetylcholine receptor antibodies were negative and creatine kinase (CK) was raised at 482. Genetic testing revealed an expansion in the first exon of the polyadenylation binding protein nuclear 1 (PABPN1) gene, confirming a diagnosis of oculopharyngeal muscular dystrophy in both this woman and her father.

DOI: 10.1201/9780429429323-25

DIAGNOSIS

Oculopharyngeal muscular dystrophy.

Discussion

Oculopharyngeal muscular dystrophy (OPMD) is typically a late-onset genetic muscle disease presenting with ptosis, dysphagia and a degree of proximal weakness affecting all four limbs, usually in the fifth or sixth decade. It is caused by the expansion (of variable size) of GCN triplets coding for alanine in the first exon of the polyadenylation binding protein nuclear 1 (PABPN1) gene. It is possible that the gain in function of this protein, which is a ubiquitous polyadenylation factor shuttling between the nucleus and the cytoplasm forming poly-A tails in eukaryotic mRNA, leads to pathological damage but a number of hypotheses have been proposed.

The commonest form is autosomal dominant and so a number of patients have a positive family history. This form has a penetrance of <1% for carriers under 40 years old and is fully penetrant in those older than 70 years. Prevalence has been found to be highest (due to founder mutations) in a French-Canadian population in Quebec (1:1000) and in Bukhara Jews in Israel (1:600) and estimated to be 1:200,000 in France. Rarer allelic recessive forms and point mutations have also been reported. Some forms, particularly those with two autosomal dominant mutations, are more severe and present earlier, but a clear relationship between triplet repeat size and phenotype has not been established.

Most patients with OPMD have normal or mildly raised CK levels (although up to 5 times normal is reported). Myopathic changes may be evident on electromyography and dystrophic changes on muscle biopsy. Rimmed vacuoles (similar to those found in inclusion body myositis) and intranuclear inclusions of tubular filaments (containing PABPN1 and other proteins), arranged in palisades or tangles, are often seen on muscle biopsy. However, the diagnosis is usually reached by genetic testing. Genetic counselling should be made available for families.

There is currently no preventative, curative or disease-modifying therapy for OPMD. Early speech and language therapy and dietetics input are essential to manage safe swallowing and enhance nutrition. Cricopharyngeal myotomy and botulinum toxin injections to the upper oesophageal sphincter have been used to provide some relief from dysphagia, but the effects of these interventions are temporary. Gastrostomy feeding is needed in a number of cases. Cough management is important as aspiration pneumonia is a common cause of death in this patient group. Physiotherapy input will also enable a graded exercise regime, management of falls and support with mobility aids. Eyelid elevation surgery can often greatly improve the quality of life for people living with OPMD.

Learning points

- OPMD should be considered in patients with ptosis, swallowing difficulties and a limb girdle pattern of muscle weakness, particularly in cases with a positive family history.
- The differential diagnosis includes myasthenia gravis, mitochondrial myopathy (including chronic progressive external ophthalmoplegia) and myotonic dystrophy.
- Where the condition is considered, diagnosis can usually be made by genetic testing, without the need for muscle biopsy, with access to genetic counselling for families.
- Care should be taken with swallowing, nutrition and cough management. Gastrostomy feeding may needed.
- Eyelid surgery should be considered and can significantly improve quality of life.

Further reading

Bouchard JP & Barbeau A. (1997) Oculopharyngeal muscular dystrophy in French Canada and North America. *Neuromuscular Disorders* 7 (Suppl 1) S5–11 & S22–29.

Brais B. (1998) Short GCG expansions in the PABP2 gene cause oculopharyngeal muscular dystrophy. *Nature Genetics* 18(2): 164–167.

Richard P, Trollet C, Stojkovic T, de Becdelievre A, Perie S, Pouget A, Eymard B. (2017) Correlation between PABPN1 genotype and severity it oculopharyngeal muscular dystrophy. *Neurology* 88(4): 359–365.

Van der Sluijs BM, Lassche S, Knuiman GJ, Kusters B, Heerschap A, Hopman M, Schreuder TH, van Engelen BGM & Voermans NC. (2017) Involvement of pelvic girdle and proximal leg muscles in early oculopharyngeal muscular dystrophy. *Neuromuscular Disorders* 27(12): 1099–1105.

Van der Sluijs BM, Raz, V, Lammens M, van den Heuvel LP, Voermans NC & van Engelen BGM. (2016) Intranuclear aggregates precede clinical onset in oculopharyngeal muscular dystrophy. *Journal of Neuromuscular Disorders* 3(1): 101–119.

CASE 15

Stefen Brady

History

A 48-year-old man presented with a 35-year history of progressive lower limb weakness. His first symptom was difficulty climbing stairs as fast as his friends at school. At the time, he attributed this to being overweight. A few years prior to presentation, he noted increasing difficulty in lifting objects of any significant weight above shoulder height. He did not complain of any additional symptoms, including orobulbar or cardiorespiratory symptoms. His father and paternal grandmother had been similarly affected and both died in their late 70s with his grandmother requiring a wheelchair in her later years but the cause for this was unclear. He had four children, none of whom experienced any similar symptoms.

Examination

There was atrophy of his shoulder girdle muscles accompanied by mild weakness of shoulder abduction (MRC grading 4/5) and elbow flexion, and moderate weakness of hip flexion (3/5).

Investigations

His creatine kinase (CK) level was 202 IU/L (normal 40–320 IU/L). Electromyography (EMG) revealed small, short-duration polyphasic units. Muscle biopsy (Figure C15.1) demonstrated myopathic changes accompanied by the presence of large subsarcolemmal and sarcoplasmic aggregates which stained bright red on modified Gömöri trichrome staining. The aggregates were also strongly positive on nicotinamide adenine dinucleotide-tetrazolium reductase (NADH-TR) and myoadenylate deaminase (AMPDA) histochemical (HC) staining but were negative on succinate dehydrogenase (SDH) and cytochrome c oxidase (COX) HC stains. The aggregates were additionally highlighted with sarco-/endoplasmic reticulum Ca^{2+}-ATPase (SERCA1) immunohistochemical (IHC) staining. Electron microscopy of the muscle confirmed the presence of tubules within the muscle fibres (Figure C15.2).

DOI: 10.1201/9780429429323-26

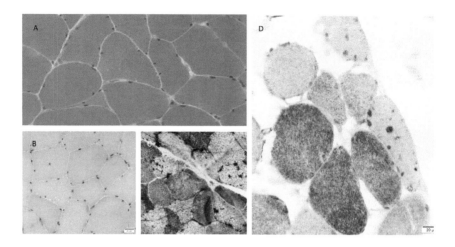

Figure C15.1 (A) Haematoxylin and eosin stain reveals mild muscle fibre size variation and atrophy. Occasional fibres showing irregular internal slits or holes (40×). (B) Modified Gömöri trichrome stain shows small slits and vacuoles in fibres, which frequently contain red material (40×). (C) The material within the slits and vacuoles is strongly positive on nicotinamide adenine dinucleotide (NADH) histochemical stain (40×). (D) sarco-/endoplasmic reticulum Ca^{2+}-ATPase (SERCA1) immunohistochemical stain highlights positive staining within the slits and vacuoles (40×).

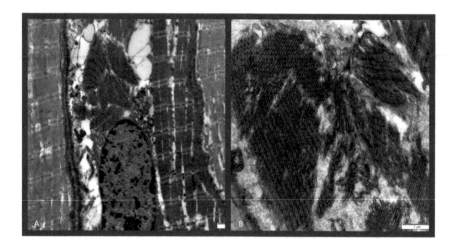

Figure C15.2 (A) Electron microscopy (EM) demonstrating the presence of 70 to 400 nm tubules with central dense material in muscle fibres (2 μm). (B) Structure of tubules visualised at greater magnification (1 μm).

DIAGNOSIS

Tubular aggregate myopathy (TAM).

Discussion

Tubular aggregates (TAs) are a distinctive histopathological feature with a characteristic staining profile. They are observed in 0.5% of muscle biopsies (1). Ultrastructural studies show they comprise clusters of closely apposed tubules and attempts to categorise them morphologically have been made (2). TAs appear as non-specific aggregates within muscle fibres on routine haematoxylin and eosin (H&E) stains. Ancillary HC and IHC staining is required to confirm the presence of the TAs, which stain red on modified Gömöri trichrome staining and are strongly positive on NADH-TR and AMPDA staining. They do not stain on other oxidative stains (SDH, COX). TAs can also be highlighted with IHC staining for SERCA1 and dysferlin and, in some patients, with SERCA2.

TAs are associated with a wide range of hereditary and acquired disorders including inflammatory, metabolic and toxic myopathies. Their aetiology is uncertain, but it is accepted that they are related to the sarcoplasmic reticulum (SR) and the result of disordered calcium homeostasis. Tubular aggregate myopathies (TAMs) are a clinically heterogeneous group of presumed hereditary disorders distinguished by the presence of prominent TAs on muscle biopsy. Four clinical phenotypes are included under the term "TAM": exertional myalgia, limb girdle myopathy, periodic paralysis and congenital myasthenic syndrome (CMS).

Although the underlying genetic cause of each phenotype of TAM is uncertain, clinical presentation and investigations can guide molecular genetic investigation and diagnosis. For example, a diagnosis of CMS with TAs is suggested by symptoms and signs of fatigability and neurophysiological evidence of a neuromuscular junction disorder. Currently, pathogenic variants in three genes are associated with CMS with TAs: *GFPT1*, *DPAGT1* and *ALG2*. In contrast, the presence of ophthalmic and haematological abnormalities, including miosis, thrombocytopenia and asplenia, are indicative of TAM associated with pathogenic variants in *STIM1* and *ORAI1*, genes that encode proteins involved in calcium homeostasis.

Finally, the size and staining characteristics of TAs in muscle can aid diagnosis (1, 3). Larger TAs in both type I and II muscle fibres are indicative of TAM, whereas smaller TAs exclusively observed in type II fibres are usually a secondary phenomenon associated with acquired disorders. The H&E staining characteristics of TAs, the electron microscopy appearances and the appearance of TAs on SERCA2 IHC staining may guide the clinician in distinguishing between forms of TAMs (3).

Learning points

- TAs are derived from the SR and have a distinctive histopathological appearance on muscle biopsy.

- TAs are associated with a wide range of acquired and hereditary disorders.
- TAMs are a heterogeneous group of hereditary disorders in which TAs are prominent.
- Clinical features such as fatigability and miosis and staining characteristics on muscle biopsy may aid in the diagnosis of particular TAMs and can be used to direct molecular genetic testing for known genes involved in TAMs.

Further reading

1. Funk F, Ceuterick-de Groote C, Martin JJ, et al. Morphological spectrum and clinical features of myopathies with tubular aggregates. *Histol Histopathol*. 2013;28:1041–54.
2. Pavlovicová M, Novotová M, Zahradník I. Structure and composition of tubular aggregates of skeletal muscle fibres. *Gen Physiol Biophys*. 2003;22:425–40.
3. Brady S, Healy EG, Gang Q, et al. Tubular aggregates and cylindrical spirals have distinct immunohistochemical signatures. *J Neuropathol Exp Neurol*. 2016;75:1171–8.

Case 16

Andria Merrison

PATIENT ASSESSMENT

History

A 32-year-old woman presented with a 4-year history of progressive proximal weakness in all four limbs, with difficulty rising from a seated position, carrying shopping bags and unsteadiness on climbing stairs. She also reported mild swallowing difficulties and a degree of muscle stiffness, particularly in the hands on cold days. She had had surgery for cataracts in her late 20s, had ongoing problems with abdominal pain, and had both significant sleep disruption and excessive daytime sleepiness. In recent months she had found that she fell asleep whenever she sat down to rest in the day.

Examination

On examination, there was frontal balding, bilateral ptosis, and facial and neck weakness. There was weakness grade 4+/5 of shoulder abduction and hip flexion (with some wasting of the quadricep muscles bilaterally). Grip and percussion myotonia was evident in both hands.

Investigations

Routine blood tests, including creatine kinase (CK), were normal. An abdominal ultrasound revealed faecal loading and gallstones. An electrocardiogram (ECG) demonstrated first-degree heart block. Lung function tests showed a forced vital capacity (FVC) of 45% of predicted and multiple dips in oxygenation overnight.

DIAGNOSIS

Myotonic dystrophy type 1 (DM1).

Discussion

Myotonic dystrophy (DM1) is the most common form of adult-onset muscular dystrophy, with prevalence of 3–15/100,000. It is an autosomal dominant progressive multisystem disorder due to an expansion of an unstable trinucleotide repeat (CTG) sequence in the myotonic dystrophy protein kinase (DPMK) gene on chromosome 19q13.3. The DPMK gene codes for myotonin protein kinase, a myosin kinase found in skeletal muscle. DM1 demonstrates genetic anticipation: increasing severity and decreasing age of onset in successive generations (which also correlates with the length of the CTG repeat sequence). Most patients present in adult life, but those with larger repeats may present in childhood and a severe (sometimes fatal) congenital form arises when a mother with a moderate-sized expansion passes on a large expansion to a fetus.

DM1 typically presents with distal onset weakness and myotonia (failure of muscle relaxation after contraction) with proximal progression. Ptosis, facial weakness, neck weakness (particularly sternocleidomastoid), fatigue, dysphagia, gallstones, gastrointestinal dysmotility, frontal balding and early cataracts are common. A number of endocrine abnormalities are also associated with DM1: impaired glucose tolerance, thyroid and hypothalamic dysfunction, testicular atrophy (with male infertility) and menstrual irregularities.

Respiratory complications are multifactorial: obstructive sleep apnoea (OSA), respiratory muscle weakness and central apnoea. Respiratory failure (with diaphragmatic and intercostal muscle weakness), usually with aspiration pneumonia (due to a weak cough), is the commonest cause of early mortality in DM1. Patients with DM1 may have increased sensitivity to drugs that depress ventilator drive (including opiates, barbiturates and anaesthetic agents) making planning of anaesthesia important.

Cardiac rhythm disturbance, particularly conduction disturbances and tachyarrhythmias are also common and contribute significantly to morbidity and mortality, accounting for 30% of deaths in patients with DM1. Cardiomyopathy is rarely a feature of DM1.

Fatigue or excessive daytime sleepiness occurs in 40% of patients with DM1 and can have a profound effect on quality of life. Respiratory failure (particularly hypercapnia) needs to be excluded as a cause, but it more commonly arises as part of central nervous system dysfunction. Cognitive and intellectual deficits are frequent in adult-onset DM1 but are usually much milder than in those with congenital or childhood-onset forms. A range of psychiatric complications are reported. Apathy, depression and anxiety are experienced by many with DM1.

The diagnosis can only be confirmed by DNA analysis. Myotonia may be detected on electromyography. Patients should be screened for complications, with regular screening for respiratory and cardiac complications in particular.

Management and treatment require multidisciplinary support from a range of therapy services. Continuous positive airway pressure (CPAP) ventilation may be used to treat OSA and bilevel positive airway pressure (BiPAP) for respiratory muscle weakness/central apnoea. A number of patients are unable to tolerate non-invasive ventilation. A pacemaker or implantable cardioverter defibrillator may be required for cardiac rhythm disturbances. Modafinil may be helpful in treating excessive daytime sleepiness and mexiletine may alleviate myotonia. Gene therapy, including development of antisense molecules that will reduce mutant DPMK, offers potential hope for disease-modifying therapies in DM1.

Learning points
- DM1 is the commonest form of adult-onset muscular dystrophy.
- DM1 is a multisystem disorder with a wide range of neurological and other medical complications, including diabetes, hypothyroidism and early cataracts.
- Respiratory and cardiac complications are common causes of morbidity and mortality, requiring lifelong screening and appropriate intervention.

Further reading
Ashizawa T et al. 2019. Consensus-based care recommendations for adults with myotonic dystrophy type 1. *Neurology Clinical Practice* 8(6): 507–520.

Catalano A, Franchini C & Carocci A. 2021. Voltage-gated sodium channel blockers: synthesis of mexiletine analogues and homologues. *Current Medicinal Chemistry* 28(8): 1535–1548.

Gonzalez-Alegre P 2019. Recent advances in molecular therapies in neurological disease: triplet repeat disorders. *Human Molecular Genetics* 28(R1): R80–87.

McNally EM, Mann DL, Pinto Y, Bakhta D, Tomiselli G, Nazarian S, Groh WJ, Tamura T, Duboc D, Itoh H, Hellerstein L & Mammen PPA 2020. Clinical care recommendations for cardiologists treating adults with myotonic dystrophy. *Journal of the American Heart Association* 9(4): e014006. doi: 10.1161/JAHA.119.014006

Stoodley J, Vallejo-Bedia F, Seone-Miraz D, Debasa-Mouce, Wood MJA & Varela MA 2023. Application of antisense conjugates for the treatment of myotonic dystrophy type 1. *International Journal of Molecular Sciences* 24(3): 2697.

Thornton CA, Wymer JP, Simmons Z, McClain C, Moxley RT. 1997. Expansion of the myotonic dystrophy CTG repeat reduces expression of the flanking DMAHP gene. *Nature Genetics* 16: 407–1409.

Timchenko L 2022. Development of therapeutic approaches for myotonic dystrophies type 1 and type 2. *International Journal of Molecular Sciences* 23(18): 10491.

CASE 17

Andria Merrison

History

A 30-year-old man presented with a 2-year history of progressive weakness in the lower limbs, with increasing difficulty rising from a seated position. He had also begun to notice mild weakness in the upper limbs when carrying heavy bags or moving furniture. He reported daily muscle pain and stiffness, including difficulty releasing his hand grip at times, which was a little worse in hot weather.

He did not report any other neurological symptoms and had been systemically well.

His mother had been similarly affected by lower limb weakness, muscle pain and stiffness. She had started walking with a stick at the age of 48.

Examination

On examination, there was evidence of thinning of the quadriceps muscle bilaterally, without fasciculation, and hip flexion weakness grade 4+5. He had bilateral calf hypertrophy. Elbow extension was also mildly weak (4++/5). There was evidence of both grip and percussion myotonia in the hands bilaterally. Reflexes were present and symmetrical and plantars flexor.

He had mild sensorineural hearing impairment but all other cranial nerves were intact and sensory examination was normal.

Investigations

Creatine kinase (CK) was raised at 676 U/L. HbA1C was mildly raised at 44 mmol/mol.

An electrocardiogram (ECG) showed first-degree heart block.

Electromyography revealed myotonic discharges and myopathic changes in multiple muscle groups.

Genetic testing established the diagnosis.

 DOI: 10.1201/9780429429323-28

DIAGNOSIS

Myotonic dystrophy type 2 (DM2).

Discussion

Myotonic dystrophy type 2 (DM2, previously known as proximal myotonic myopathy [PROMM]) is a multisystem autosomal dominant disorder characterised by myotonia, proximal weakness early in the course of the disease, and often myalgia and fatigue. Myotonia may be identified clinically (grip and percussion myotonia) and with electromyography (EMG). Creatine kinase may be mildly elevated (<10 times the upper limit of normal).

With an estimated prevalence of 2 per 100,000, DM2 is much less common than DM1 and most families with this condition are from Northern Europe. It usually presents in adulthood, in the third decade, and although infrequently reported in children. It typically causes neck/axial, elbow extension and hip flexion weakness at onset. If distal muscles are affected, this tends to occur later in the disease course, and unlike DM1, facial weakness and dysphagia are uncommon (Table C17.1).

Systemic features include cardiac conduction defects (20%), posterior subcapsular cataracts, sensorineural hearing impairment (60%), insulin insensitivity, testicular failure, hyperhidrosis, gastrointestinal disturbance, obstructive sleep apnoea and rarely respiratory failure. Magnetic resonance imaging identifies white matter changes in over 50% of patients (as well as reduced frontal, parietal, thalamic and/or hippocampal grey matter reduction in some). However, cognitive difficulties tend to be much less severe in DM2 than in DM1. Cardiac (annual ECG) and respiratory monitoring (at baseline and in the context of symptoms) are recommended, as well as screening for other systemic complications.

DM2 is caused by an unstable CCTG repeat sequence expansion in intron 1 of the cellular nucleic binding protein (CNBP, previously known as the zinc finger binding protein gene [ZNF9]) on chromosome 3q21.3. The expansion ranges from 75 to 11,000 repeats, and unlike DM1, the size of the repeat does not closely correlate with age of onset or disease severity. The repeat sequence disrupts muscle chloride channel RNA, which in turn leads to myotonia. Zinc binding protein is found in greatest abundance in skeletal and cardiac muscle in both the cytoplasm and on the endoplasmic reticulum. It is involved in the translation of ornithine decarboxylase mRNA and in sterol-mediated transcriptional regulation.

Whilst there are currently no curative treatments for DM2, supportive therapy (treatment of complications, physiotherapy, occupational therapy, psychological support and genetic counselling) can be beneficial. As primary disorders of RNA splicing mechanisms, DM2 and DM1 have the potential to be treated or modified by gene therapies.

Table C17.1 Comparative features of myotonic dystrophy type 1 (DM1) and type 2 (DM2)

Feature	DM1	DM2
Gene	DMPK	CNBP
Chromosome	19q13.3	3q.21
Mutation type	CTG repeat	CCTG repeat
Repeat size	50–4000	Mean in 1000s
Age of onset	Any	Adulthood mainly
Anticipation	Yes	Not usually
Congenital form	Yes	Rarely
Facial/neck weakness, dysphagia	Common	Uncommon
Weak limbs, proximal	Late	Early
Weak limbs, distal	Early	Late
Myotonia	Mild to moderate	Mild to moderate
Electromyography myotonia	Very common	Common
Myalgia	Mild to moderate	Mild to severe
Cataracts	Very common/early	Common
Frontal balding	Very common	Uncommon
Cardiac dysrhythmia	Very common/early	Common/late
Respiratory failure	Very common/late	Uncommon
Cognitive dysfunction	Common/mild to severe	Uncommon
Gonadal failure	Common	Uncommon
Excessive daytime sleepiness	Very common/early	Common/late
Hyperhidrosis	Mild	Mild to severe

Learning points

- Myotonic dystrophy type 2 is a multisystem autosomal dominant disorder, characterised by myotonia and progressive proximal weakness, usually presenting in the third decade of life.
- Cardiac conduction defects, respiratory compromise, sensorineural deafness, cataracts and other systemic complications can arise.
- Myotonic dystrophy type 2 is much less common than myotonic dystrophy but shares a number of features. Early distal weakness and cognitive problems are much less common in myotonic dystrophy type 2 than in myotonic dystrophy type 1.
- Whilst there are no disease-modifying treatments currently available, as a disorder of RNA splicing mechanisms, gene therapy may offer hope for the future.

Further reading

Hamel J, McDermott MP, Hilbert JE, Martens WB, Luebbe E, Tawil R, Moxley JT & Thornton CA (2022) Milestones of progression in myotonic dystrophy type 1 and type 2. *Muscle & Nerve* 66(4): 508–512.

Ivanovic V, Peric S, Pesovic J, Tubic R, Bozovic I, Petrovic Djordjevic I, Savic-Pavicevic D, Meola G & Rakocevic-Stojanovic V (2022) Clinical score for early diagnosis of myotonic dystrophy type 2. *Neurological Sciences* Nov 19. doi: 10.1007/s10072-022-06507-9.

LoRusso S, Weiner B & Arnold WD (2018) Myotonic dystrophies: targeting therapies in multisystem disease. *Neurotherapeutics* 15(4): 872–884.

Meola G. (2020) Myotonic dystrophy type 2: the 2020 update. *Acta Myologica* 39(4): 222–234.

Roy B, Wu Q, Whitaker CH & Felice KJJ (2021) Myotonic muscular dystrophy type 2 in CT, USA: a single centre experience with 50 patients. *Journal of Clinical Neuromuscular Disease* 22(3): 135–146.

Udd B, Krahe R, Wallgren-Pettersson C, Falck B & Kalimo H (1997) Proximal myotonic dystrophy – a family with autosomal dominant muscular dystrophy, cataracts, hearing loss and hypogonadism: heterogeneity of proximal myotonic syndromes? *Neuromuscular Disorders* 7: 217–228.

CASE 18

Andria Merrison

History

A 24-year-old presented with generalised muscle stiffness, which at times was uncomfortable, and intermittent weakness in the legs. He had always had very well-developed musculature but had sometimes struggled with sport at school.

He was working as a builder and reported that if he was working some distance from home his muscles would get stiffer and his legs feel weak when he first stepped out of the van. Once he got working these symptoms would improve and he was able to labour throughout the day. His symptoms were sometimes a little worse on a cold day but not markedly so.

He did not report any other neurological symptoms. Other than mild asthma as a child, he did not have any other significant medical problems and was not taking any medication.

Examination

On examination, there was generalised muscle hypertrophy. There was hand grip myotonia and percussion myotonia in the thenar eminence bilaterally. The neurological examination was otherwise normal and power was preserved in all muscle groups.

Investigations

Creatine kinase (CK) was raised at 893 U/l.

Electromyography (EMG) demonstrated early decrement in compound muscle action potentials (CMAPs) with rapid recovery. Cooling did not alter these changes. Frequent myotonic discharges were seen, particularly in the lower limbs.

DOI: 10.1201/9780429429323-29

DIAGNOSIS

Myotonia congenita.

Discussion

Myotonia congenita is a rare genetic condition, with an estimated prevalence of 1–7/100,000, caused by mutations in the chloride channel gene CLCN1. It is a channelopathy due to dysfunction of an ion channel, voltage-gated chloride channel, present in the muscle sarcolemma and one of a group of conditions identified as non-dystrophic myotonias. Other non-dystrophic myotonias include paramyotonia congenita and sodium channel myotonia (including potassium and cold-aggravated myotonias). Myotonia congenita is the only muscle channelopathy known to be inherited in either a recessive (Becker disease) or a dominant (Thomson disease) form.

Whilst the age of onset of myotonia congenita is usually in the first decade, there is a wide spectrum of presentation from the first to the fourth decade. The severity and distribution of myotonia varies, but it is often most marked in the lower limbs. Muscle hypertrophy can be very significant and may be overlooked in younger patients who are very active.

Myotonia in this condition typically demonstrates the "warm-up phenomenon" where symptoms improve with repetitive muscle action and are often worst after a period of rest, including transient weakness. A cold environment may exacerbate myotonia, but this is much less common than in patients with paramyotonia congenita. Myotonia may be seen by examining for lid lag (myotonia of orbicularis oculi more commonly seen in paramyotonia congenita), hand grip and percussion of the thenar eminence. In all non-dystrophic myotonias, proximal myopathy may develop over time. Unlike myotonic dystrophy, other systemic features are not associated with non-dystrophic myotonia.

CK may be raised (usually less than 1000 U/l) but may be normal. Electromyography reveals myotonic discharges and a fall in CMAP, reflecting initial muscle weakness, that rapidly recovers with each repetition, reflecting improvement in muscle strength. This short exercise test can be used, including at different temperatures, to distinguish forms of non-dystrophic myotonia. Genetic testing is diagnostic and may require sequencing of the whole CLCN1 gene.

There are currently no drugs that directly target the dysfunctional chloride channel. However, mexiletine (a sodium channel blocker, including the SCN4A channel, used in sodium channelopathies and paramyotonia congenita) is the most effective and well-tolerated form of treatment for myotonia in this condition. Its use has now been supported by two randomised controlled trials in non-dystrophic myotonia. Flecainide, propafenone, lamotrigine and acetazolamide have all been used to ameliorate symptoms. Gene-modifying therapies may well form future treatment for myotonia congenita.

Learning points

- Myotonia congenita is channelopathy caused by mutations in the voltage-gated chloride channel gene CLCN1, which can be autosomal recessive (Becker disease) or dominant (Thomson disease).
- Myotonia in this condition demonstrates the "warm-up phenomenon" where myotonia improves with exercise and is worst when trying to move after a period of rest.
- Muscle hypertrophy can easily be overlooked in young people who are very physically active, but muscle stiffness and sometimes proximal muscle weakness are present in the context of well-developed musculature.
- EMG usually demonstrates early decrement in CMAPs and widespread myotonic discharges.
- Mexiletine (a cardiac antiarrhythmic sodium channel blocker) is the most effective and well-tolerated treatment for myotonia in this condition.

Further reading

Jitpimolmard N, Matthews E & Fialho D (2020) Treatment updates for neuromuscular channelopathies. *Current Treatment Options Neurology* 22(10): 34.

Statland JM, Bundy BN, Wang Y, Rayan DR, Trivedi JR, Sansone VA et al. (2012) Mexiletine for symptoms and signs of myotonia in non-dystrophic myotonia: a randomised controlled trial. *JAMA* 308:1357–1365.

Stunnenberg BC, LoRusso S, Arnold WD, Barohn RJ, Cannon SC, Fontaine B, Griggs RC, Hanna MG, Matthews E, Meola G, Sansone VA, Trivedi JR, van Engelen BGM, Vicart S, Statland JM. (2020) Guidelines on clinical presentation and management of non-dystrophic myotonias. *Muscle and Nerve* 62(4):430–444.

Stunnenberg BC, Raaphorst J, Groenewoud HM, Statland JM, Griggs RC, Woertman W, et al. (2018) Effect of mexiletine on muscle stiffness in patients with nondystrophic myotonia evaluated using aggregated N-of-1 trials. *JAMA* 320:2344–2353.

Vivekanandam V, Jaibaji R, Sud R, Ellmers R, Skorupinska I, Germaine L, James N, Holmes S, Mannikko R, Jayaseelan D, Hanna MG. (2023) Prevalence of genetically confirmed skeletal muscle channelopathies in the era of next generation sequencing. *Neuromuscular Disorders* 33(3):270–273.

Vivekanandam V, Munot P, Hanna MG, Matthews E. (2020) Skeletal muscle channelopathies. *Neurologic Clinics.* 8(3):481–491.

CASE 19

Stefen Brady

PATIENT ASSESSMENT

History

An 84-year-old Caucasian woman was referred with a 3-year history of progressive difficulty picking up small objects, which had been initially attributed to osteoarthritis. She described her hands as being weak and uncomfortable. For many years, she struggled to rise from low chairs but believed this was normal for her age. She had recently fallen several times, which she had also attributed to her age. On direct questioning, she admitted to mild dysphagia unaccompanied by disturbance of speech. Her previous medical history included osteoarthritis, gout, bilateral hearing loss and hypertension. She took allopurinol and enalapril daily. She had no family history of note.

Examination

There was mild bilateral periocular facial weakness and mild weakness (MRC grading 4/5) of neck flexion. Scalloping of the volar (anterior) forearm muscles was also identified along with asymmetric mild weakness (4/5) of shoulder abduction and elbow extension, and the inability to make a fist with either hand (illustrative picture in a male patient Figure C19.1A). Lower limb examination revealed bilateral atrophy of the quadriceps muscles (illustrative picture in a male patient Figure C19.1B) with moderate asymmetric weakness (3/5) of hip flexion, knee extension and ankle dorsiflexion.

Investigations

Her creatine kinase (CK) level was normal (49 IU/L; normal 25–200 IU/L). Nerve conduction studies (NCS) were normal. Electromyography (EMG) revealed positive sharp waves and small, short-duration, polyphasic motor units. A muscle biopsy from the deltoid muscle showed a combination of inflammatory and myopathic changes with significant variation of muscle fibre size observed (comprising a combination of both rounded and angulated atrophic fibres admixed with occasional hypertrophic fibres), perimysial and endomysial mononuclear inflammation (including invasion of intact muscle fibres, also referred to as partial invasion), rimmed vacuoles (vacuoles within muscle fibres surrounded by granular deposits), increased mitochondrial changes, upregulation of expression of sarcolemmal major histocompatibility complex class I (MHC class I), and p62-immunohistochemical staining identified sarcolemmal aggregates.

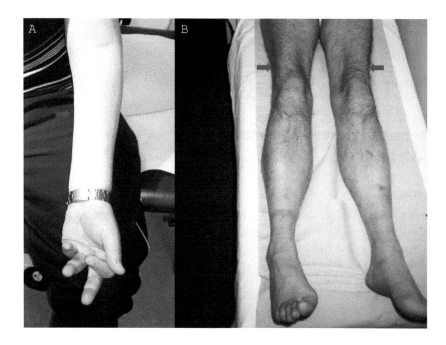

Figure C19.1 (A) Scalloping or concavity of the medial (ulnar) aspect of the forearm indicative of atrophy of the volar forearm muscles (arrow) in a male patient and the patient attempting to make a closed fist. (B) Marked bilateral atrophy of the distal quadriceps muscles in a male patient (arrows).

DIAGNOSIS

Inclusion body myositis (IBM).

Discussion

Inclusion body myositis (IBM) is the commonest acquired myopathy in individuals over 50 years of age. It is classified as an idiopathic inflammatory myopathy (IIM) along with polymyositis and dermatomyositis, but its clinical presentation and response to treatment bear little resemblance to either of these diseases.

IBM appears to be more frequent in Caucasian populations and males are affected twice as often as females. It has a characteristic clinical presentation. Initial symptoms include difficulty rising from a chair and ascending stairs due to proximal lower limb weakness. Sudden falls are typical and result from the development of significant early weakness of the quadriceps muscles. Finger flexion weakness impairs manual dexterity and is a less frequent presenting symptom feature but may be reported. Mild dysphagia is common but is rarely the presenting complaint. The most frequent signs at presentation are knee extension weakness (greater than or equal to hip flexion weakness) and long finger flexion weakness. Other frequently affected muscles are the periocular muscles, elbow extensors, hip flexors and ankle dorsiflexors (1). Limb weakness is often asymmetric.

CK is usually mildly elevated in IBM (<1000 U/L) but can be normal or moderately raised. Values above 3000 IU/L are uncommon and should lead to the consideration of alternative diagnoses. EMG may show both neurogenic changes (fibrillations and positive sharp waves) and myopathic features. Up until the last decade, muscle biopsy was the cornerstone of diagnosis. Histopathological features classically associated with IBM include the presence of an endomysial lymphocytic infiltrate with inflammatory cells invading intact muscle fibres (partial invasion), rimmed vacuoles, and 15–18 nm tubulofilamentous inclusions on electron microscopy or muscle fibre amyloid (Figure C19.2). Although these histopathological findings together are highly specific for IBM, they lack sensitivity, and ultrastructural studies and amyloid staining are infrequently performed. Additional histopathological features which, when present in an inflammatory myopathy, support a diagnosis of IBM are mitochondrial changes and p62-positive aggregates (1, 2).

The pathogenesis of IBM is uncertain and currently there is no known effective treatment available (3, 4). However, an initial trial of rapamycin showed promise and a larger trial is being conducted along with other trials. Although IBM is a slowly progressive disease, it is very disabling due to the early and marked involvement of the distal upper limb and proximal lower limb muscles.

Management aims to slow deterioration through regular exercise and to maximise function with the use of aids. Dysphagia is successfully managed by most individuals with IBM. However, for some individuals with IBM, it is a significant problem contributing to malnutrition, social phobia and aspiration pneumonia.

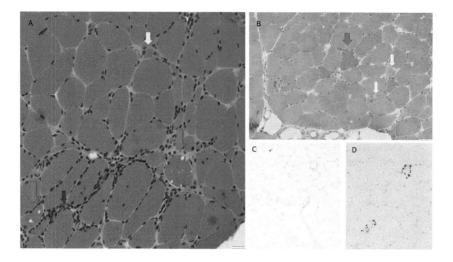

Figure C19.2 Inclusion Body Myositis muscle biopsy. (A) Haematoxylin and eosin stain demonstrating an endomysial inflammatory infiltrate (purple arrow), vacuoles within muscle fibres (blue arrows), and necrotic fibres (yellow arrow) (20×). (B) Modified Gömöri trichrome showing rimmed vacuoles (blue arrow) and scattered necrotic fibres (yellow arrows) (20×). (C) Major histocompatibility complex (MHC) class 1 immunohistochemical (IHC) stain highlighting diffuse increased sarcolemmal expression around muscle fibres (20×). (D) p62 IHC stain revealing p62-positive granular subsarcolemmal inclusions in rimmed vacuoles (40×).

In such situations, treatment options include balloon dilatation or myotomy of the cricopharyngeal muscle (if it is hypertrophied), or gastrostomy.

IBM was not thought to be significantly life limiting. However, a survey revealed that it was the primary or secondary cause of death in 40% of individuals affected by it (5). In addition, the risk of premature death was sevenfold higher among those persons with IBM.

Learning points

- IBM is the commonest acquired myopathy in individuals over 50 years of age.
- The clinical presentation of IBM is highly characteristic.
- Muscle biopsy should be considered supportive of the clinical diagnosis rather than diagnostic.
- Currently, there is no effective treatment for IBM and management is largely supportive.

Further reading

1. Brady S, Squier W, Hilton-Jones D. Clinical assessment determines the diagnosis of inclusion body myositis independently of pathological features. *Journal of Neurology, Neurosurgery & Psychiatry* 2013;84:1240–1246.

2. Brady S, Squier W, Sewry C, *et al.* A retrospective cohort study identifying the principal pathological features useful in the diagnosis of inclusion body myositis. *BMJ Open* 2014;4:e004552.
3. Rose MR; ENMC IBM Working Group. 188th ENMC International Workshop: Inclusion Body Myositis, 2-4 December 2011, Naarden, The Netherlands. *Neuromuscul Disord.* 2013;23:1044–1055.
4. Benveniste O, Guiguet M, Freebody J, *et al.* Long-term observational study of sporadic inclusion body myositis. *Brain.* 201;134:3176–3184.
5. Price MA, Barghout V, Benveniste O, *et al.* Mortality and causes of death in patients with sporadic inclusion body myositis: Survey study based on the clinical experience of specialists in Australia, Europe and the USA. *Journal of Neuromuscular Diseases* 3, 67–75.

CASE 20

Kezia Austin and Harsha Gunawardena

PATIENT ASSESSMENT

History

A 33-year-old woman presented with acute onset of muscle weakness in all four limbs, along with difficulty swallowing and voice change. These symptoms had progressed rapidly, following a 1-month prodrome of malaise and severe myalgia. She had noticed increasingly poor grip strength as well as proximal limb girdle weakness that meant she had been unable to get out of the bath or climb the stairs without assistance. She had also developed an erythematous rash over the face, back and chest. There were no joint or cardiorespiratory symptoms. Later in her clinical course, after around 18 months, she began developing hard subcutaneous lesions over the abdomen and right buttock, which gradually became more widespread affecting both buttocks, breasts, thighs, arms, spine and scapulae. Prior to the onset of these symptoms, she had been fit and well and did not take any regular medications.

Examination

On initial examination, she had widespread weakness in both proximal and distal muscle groups, including neck flexion. She was dysphonic, with evidence of mild respiratory muscle weakness on forced vital capacity testing, and had a number of skin changes including heliotrope rash, periorbital oedema, and shawl sign over the chest and upper back. She subsequently developed marked atrophy of the proximal muscles, as well as widespread calcinosis with areas of overlying ulceration and skin necrosis.

Investigations

Initial creatine kinase (CK) was 15,000 U/L (normal range 40–320 U/L), which responded to initial treatment and stabilised at 300–800 U/L in the 20 years since diagnosis. Magnetic resonance imaging demonstrated widespread muscle oedema, particularly in the gluteus maximus, vastus lateralis and vastus intermedius muscles. Initial muscle biopsy of vastus lateralis demonstrated muscle fibre necrosis, perifascicular atrophy and infiltration by inflammatory cells. Areas of infarction with pale-staining muscle fibres were seen. Some blood vessels had thickened walls. A PET-CT scan showed widespread muscle oedema as well as calcification in the subcutaneous tissues of the buttocks (Figure C20.1), but no evidence of solid organ malignancy. Some years later, myositis immunoblot confirmed the presence of anti-nuclear matrix protein-2 (anti-NXP-2) antibodies.

 DOI: 10.1201/9780429429323-31

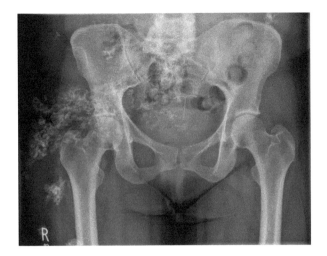

Figure C20.1 Radiograph demonstrating extensive subcutaneous calcification over the right hemipelvis and buttock.

Treatment

The patient underwent an initial 6-month admission, including extensive rehabilitation with physiotherapy and speech and language therapy. Despite an initial response to systemic immune suppression, the disease has since proven refractory to multiple treatments including glucocorticoids, methotrexate, azathioprine, tacrolimus, infliximab, intravenous immunoglobulin, mycophenolate, rituximab and cyclophosphamide. Whilst the patient's weakness and skin rashes stabilised, along with CK levels, her subcutaneous calcinosis progressed and was complicated by overlying skin ulceration and superadded infections requiring several admissions to hospital for intravenous antibiotic therapy. A low-dose intravenous cyclophosphamide regime subsequently provided stabilisation of the disease.

DIAGNOSIS

Anti-NXP-2 antibody adult-onset dermatomyositis.

Discussion

Dermatomyositis is a rare inflammatory myopathy characterised by proximal muscle weakness and typical skin changes. It affects both adults and children, and is heterogeneous in its clinical and extramuscular features, response to treatment and overall prognosis. Increasing numbers of autoantibodies have been identified in dermatomyositis patients, and these can help define individual clinical syndromes.

A novel autoantibody – originally termed anti-MJ – was identified in 1997 in a cohort of juvenile dermatomyositis patients with severe muscle weakness as well as joint contractures and gastrointestinal vasculitis.[1] The antigen was subsequently recognised as NXP-2, antibodies to which have been found in 23% of juvenile dermatomyositis patients, and strongly associates with the presence of calcinosis.[2]

Less commonly, anti-NXP-2 antibodies can also be detected in adult dermatomyositis patients, at a frequency of around 1–2%. Similar to anti-NXP-2 juvenile-onset disease, adult patients can also develop calcinosis alongside other hallmark clinical features. Calcinosis can be chronic, progressive and refractory to treatments despite response with other manifestations. Anti-NXP-2 adult dermatomyositis can be associated with malignancy and appears to be a cancer-associated phenotype compared to other clinic-serological subsets but not as strong as anti-TIF1 positive dermatomyositis. Interstitial lung disease is not a prevalent association.[3-6]

Although performed less, given the preference of myositis autoantibody screening, muscle biopsy shows a characteristic pattern of changes including perifascicular atrophy of myofibres combined with variable, often severe lymphocytic inflammation in the perimysium. Immunostaining typically demonstrates upregulation of inflammation markers, particularly MHC1 (which shows a gradient of staining increasing at the periphery of fascicles) and expression of C5b9 (or membrane attack complex [MAC]) on the sarcolemma of the same fibres. Expression of MXA (myxovirus resistance protein A) and type 1 interferon has now been reported on the peripheral atrophic myofibres in classic cases of dermatomyositis associated with anti-MDA5, anti-NXP-2, anti-TIF1 and anti-MI2 autoantibodies and can help differentiate dermatomyositis from other inflammatory myopathies.

Immune suppression can be successful in treating patients with dermatomyositis and minimising its complications. Glucocorticoids, methotrexate, azathioprine, mycophenolate, tacrolimus, infliximab, intravenous immunoglobulin, rituximab and cyclophosphamide have all been used to treat dermatomyositis.

Learning points

- Anti-NXP-2 dermatomyositis is more common in children but can affect adult-onset disease.
- Anti-NXP-2 dermatomyositis should be suspected in adult patients with relapsing–remitting inflammatory myopathy, refractory skin disease and evidence of progressive calcinosis.
- This condition can be difficult to manage and requires aggressive immunosuppression in order to prevent progression of calcinosis, which is associated with significant morbidity for patients.
- Autoantibody testing is helpful in identifying causative antibodies. In some cases, muscle biopsy may help confirm the diagnosis by demonstrating classical changes in the muscle.

Further reading

1. Oddis CV, Fertig N, Goel A, et al. Clinical and serological characterization of the anti-MJ antibody in childhood myositis. *Arthritis Rheum* 1997;40(9):S139.
2. Gunawardena H, Wedderburn LR, Chinoy H, et al. Autoantibodies to a 140-kd protein in juvenile dermatomyositis are associated with calcinosis. *Arthritis Rheum* 2009;60:1807–14.
3. Ichimura Y, Matsushita T, Hamaguchi Y, et al. Anti-NXP2 autoantibodies in adult patients with idiopathic inflammatory myopathies: possible association with malignancy. *Ann Rheum Dis*. 2012 May;71(5):710–3.
4. Albayda J, Pinal-Fernandez I, Huang W, et al. Antinuclear matrix protein 2 autoantibodies and edema, muscle disease, and malignancy risk in dermatomyositis patients. *Arthritis Care Res (Hoboken)* 2017;69(11):1771–76.
5. Fiorentino DF, Chung LS, Christopher-Stine L, et al. Most patients with cancer-associated dermatomyositis have antibodies to nuclear matrix protein NXP-2 or transcription intermediary factor 1gamma. *Arthritis Rheum* 2013;65:2954–62.
6. Linqing Zhong, Zhongxun Yu, Hongmei Song. Association of anti-nuclear matrix protein 2 antibody with complications in patients with idiopathic inflammatory myopathies: A meta-analysis of 20 cohorts. *Clin Immunol* 2019;198:11–18.

CASE 21

Charlotte David and Joel David

PATIENT ASSESSMENT

History

A 59-year-old ex-smoker of 40 pack-years presented with a 5-week history of cough and shortness of breath. He had arthralgia of the hands, wrists and shoulders with accompanying morning stiffness. His brother has systemic lupus erythematosus (SLE). There was no pet or asbestos exposure.

Examination

He was apyrexial and normotensive with shortness of breath on exertion and oxygen saturation of 93% on air. Chest examination revealed bi-basal crepitations. His hands were swollen particularly at the MCP and PIP joints, as well as the wrists. There was rough skin with some peeling at the fingertips. There was mild tenderness of the proximal muscles with a suggestion of weak resisted neck flexion and hip flexors (MRC grade 4/5).

Investigations

Full blood count revealed a white cell count of 11×10^9/L (normal range 4–10) and neutrophil count of 7.6×10^9/L (normal range 2–7). The C-reactive protein (CRP) was 86 and creatine kinase (CK) was 2192 (20–220 U/L). The chest x-ray was consistent with ground glass changes and a possible superimposed infection. The high-resolution computed tomography (HRCT) was consistent with non-specific interstitial pneumonitis (NSIP), namely, ground glass opacification, reticulation and traction bronchiectasis. The autoantibody profile was ANA positive with Jo-1 antibody positive. Magnetic resonance imaging (MRI) of the upper legs showed mild STIR hyperintensity of the left rectus femoris muscle and, to a lesser extent, left vastus, intermedius and lateralis. A muscle biopsy from the vastus lateralis demonstrated macrophage-predominant perimysial inflammation with perifascicular and myopathic changes, including muscle fibre atrophy and regeneration with scattered muscle fibre necrosis.

 DOI: 10.1201/9780429429323-32

DIAGNOSIS

Anti-Jo-1–positive antisynthetase syndrome.

Treatment and outcome

Initially, empirical antibiotics were given to cover a possible chest infection. Intravenous (IV) methylprednisolone 500 mg was administered on 3 consecutive days and cyclophosphamide 1 g fortnightly for three doses and thereafter every 3 weeks for a further three doses. This was followed by mycophenolate mofetil 1 g twice daily (BD).

Pulmonary remission (based on HRCT) and clinical and biochemical muscle remission were achieved by 5 months. Six months later, however, the CK rose to 1980 U/L. The patient was given rituximab 1 g IV and a further pulse 2 weeks later. Mycophenolate mofetil was reduced to 750 mg BD, and methotrexate 15 mg subcutaneously weekly was added with a reducing prednisolone schedule.

Discussion

Antisythetase syndrome (ASyS) is a multisystem autoimmune disease, characterised by the presence of aminoacyl transfer RNA synthetase antibodies, most commonly anti-Jo-1. ASyS is rare and accounts for approximately 30% of inflammatory myopathies, more than 50% of which are women with a mean age of 50 years at diagnosis. Clinical manifestations, illustrated in the case described, are interstitial lung disease (ILD), myositis, arthralgia/arthritis, Raynaud's phenomenon, rashes (Gottron's papules and heliotrope rash, as seen in dermatomyositis), mechanic's hands (rough skin with cracking and peeling at the fingertips and along the side of the fingers) and fever. Prognosis and survival rates in ASyS are largely dependent on the antibody identified. Anti-PL7–positive or anti-PL12–positive patients carry a worse prognosis than those who are anti-Jo1 positive. This is due to the isolated ILD presentation of the disease, which is the main cause of mortality in ASyS patients.

Pathogenesis

The pathogenesis of ASyS is largely unknown. Like other idiopathic inflammatory myopathies (IMM), it is thought to be mediated by interferon-alpha (IFN-α) and cytokines (IL-6/IL-8/anti-TNF-α). Muscle fibre damage releases aminoacyl transfer RNA synthetases, which may trigger activation of the innate and adaptive immune system, which then targets muscle tissue.

Genetics plays a role in its association with HLA haplotypes, such as DRB1*03:01. and environmental factors, such as smoking, are also believed to be involved in the pathogenesis.

Clinical manifestations

There are two main classification criteria proposed for the diagnosis of ASyS: one by Connors et al. (2010) and the other by Solomon et al. (2011). Both criteria require the presence of an aminoacyl transfer RNA synthetase antibody.

Connors et al. (2010)	Solomon et al. (2011)
Presence of an aminoacyl transfer RNA synthetase antibody plus one or more of the following: • Raynaud's phenomenon • Arthritis • ILD • Fever (not attributable to another cause) • Mechanic's hands*	Presence of an aminoacyl transfer RNA synthetase antibody plus two major or one major and two minor criteria: Major: • ILD (not attributable to another cause) • Polymyositis or dermatomyositis Minor: • Arthritis • Raynaud's phenomenon • Mechanic's hands*

* Mechanic's hands refer to thick, cracked skin predominately on the fingertips.

The classic triad of ASyS is ILD, myositis and arthritis, however, it is more common for patients to present with an isolated manifestation, with ILD being the most common and serious of the triad. Over time, only half of patients develop the complete triad.

Investigations and findings

Autoantibodies. Several autoantibodies (anti-Jo-1, anti-PL7, anti-PL12, anti-EJ, anti-KS, anti-YRS, anti-Zo) target amino acids related to RNA synthetase (involved in protein synthesis). The antibody level can fluctuate concordantly with disease activity. Anti-Jo-1 is most prevalent and has a greater association with arthritis. It also carries a better prognosis, possibly due to earlier diagnosis. Anti-PL7 and anti-PL12 are associated with severe interstitial lung disease.

Respiratory investigations. Given the prevalence of ILD in ASyS, the following investigations are recommended at baseline as a biomarker for disease progression.

- HRCT: Patterns of changes on CT in keeping with NSIP or less commonly, organising pneumonia (mainly consolidation) initially, which may later fibrose.
- Lung function tests: Display a restrictive picture (total lung capacity <80% predicted) with a reduced diffusion capacity.
- Transthoracic echocardiography: Pulmonary hypertension can develop secondary to ILD and carries a worse prognosis.

Muscle investigations and biomarkers.

- CK: elevated.
- Electromyography (EMG): The role of EMG is limited in typical ASyS but can be used to identify a suitable area for biopsy.

- Muscle biopsy: This is not routinely performed but may be helpful when the diagnosis is not clear-cut. The typical findings include perifascicular necrosis and lack of endomysial mononuclear cellular infiltration into non-necrotic fibres (a feature present in other myopathies such as inclusion body myositis).
- MRI: This can be used to support the diagnosis through identification of changes consistent with muscle oedema.
- Both EMG and MRI can be used as biomarkers. CK is also helpful in monitoring disease activity, however, in chronic disease, it may be less sensitive due to the loss of muscle mass associated with advanced disease (Chatterjee et al. 2013).

Joint investigations

Ultrasonography (US): Imitates features of rheumatoid arthritis, mainly joint effusions, synovial hypertrophy and tenosynovitis.

Management

Management involves a multidisciplinary approach, namely, respiratory physicians and rheumatologists. First-line treatment for both lung and muscle manifestations involves corticosteroids with an adjunctive steroid-sparing agent (such as azathioprine, methotrexate or mycophenolate mofetil) to avoid recurrence upon weaning steroids. Add-on therapies include tacrolimus and rescue therapies include rituximab, cyclophosphamide and intravenous immunoglobulins (IVIG).

As with many immunosuppressive therapies, screening for hepatitis B and tuberculosis is required, along with avoidance of live vaccines. Patients require follow-up for medication titration, side effects and assessment of disease progression.

Learning points

- ASyS is a multisystem autoimmune disease, characterised by the presence of aminoacyl transfer RNA synthetase antibodies.
- The clinical triad of ASyS is ILD, myositis and arthritis. More commonly, it presents with an incomplete triad.
- ILD carries a high morbidity and mortality and is the main contributor to survival in ASyS.
- Diagnosis is through the presence of an aminoacyl transfer RNA synthetase antibody, in addition to clinical features.
- Baseline investigations include lung function tests and HRCT of the thorax.
- Biomarkers of disease progression include respiratory investigations, CK, EMG and muscle MRI.
- The mainstay of treatment is corticosteroids with an additional steroid-sparing agent.

Further reading

Chatterjee, S., Prayson, R. and Farver, C. Antisynthetase syndrome: not just an inflammatory myopathy. *Cleve Clin J Med*, 2013; 80(10):655–666.

Connors GR, Christopher-Stine L, Oddis CV, Danoff SK. Interstitial lung disease associated with the idiopathic inflammatory myopathies: What progress has been made in the past 35 years? *Chest.* 2010;138:1464–1474.

Solomon J, Swigris JJ, Brown KK. Myositis-related interstitial lung disease and antisynthetase syndrome. *Jornal brasileiro de pneumologia.* 2011;37:100–109.

CASE 22

Matthew Wells and Harsha Gunawardena

PATIENT ASSESSMENT

History
A 58-year-old woman presented with 6 months of fatigue, anorexia, weight loss and intermittent night sweats. This was followed by the development of myalgia and a progressive sensation of heavy, stiff legs and altered peripheral sensation. She had a dry cough and easy bruising.

Examination
Examination revealed normal muscle bulk and power with no significant muscle tenderness to palpation. Both ankle reflexes and the right knee reflex were absent. Sensation was reduced to light touch and pinprick in a glove and stocking distribution with preserved joint position and vibration sensation. Cardiorespiratory and abdominal examinations were normal.

Investigations
Blood tests showed anaemia, lymphopaenia, deranged liver function tests with raised alkaline phosphatase, preserved renal function and significantly elevated C-reactive protein. Creatine kinase was very mildly elevated (323 U/L; upper limit of normal 200U/L), and there was mild but persistent hypercalcaemia (2.70–2.80 mmol/L). Autoimmune connective tissue disease screen demonstrated negative ANA, cANCA was positive but PR3/MPO specificities were negative. Serum ACE was persistently elevated at >100 IU/L. Urinalysis revealed proteinuria and haematuria. Subsequent renal biopsy was non-diagnostic.

A CT scan of the chest, abdomen and pelvis did not show any abnormalities apart from moderate splenomegaly. PET-CT revealed diffuse avidity within the skeletal muscles without any associated chest or lymph node abnormality. EMG was non-diagnostic, and nerve conduction studies confirmed axonal sensorimotor neuropathy.

In view of the clinical presentation, a sural nerve and muscle biopsies were performed. A nerve biopsy showed chronic axonal change. The muscle biopsy revealed widespread chronic inflammatory cell infiltrate with endomysial inflammation, and perifascicular and vessel wall penetration by inflammatory cells without fibrinoid necrosis. The key diagnostic feature of the muscle biopsy was the identification of loose non-caseating granulomas. Special stains for microorganisms were negative.

DOI: 10.1201/9780429429323-33

DIAGNOSIS

Granulomatous vasculitis, clinical syndrome in keeping with sarcoidosis with myositis.

Discussion

Sarcoidosis is a heterogeneous multisystem inflammatory disorder of poorly understood aetiology. The diagnostic hallmark is granulomatous inflammation with an associated suggestive clinical syndrome. In this case, a clinical myopathy with constitutional symptoms and persistently elevated serum ACE levels, lymphopaenia, mild hypercalcaemia and splenomegaly raised early suspicion for sarcoidosis over a primary systemic vasculitis, infectious or paraneoplastic process all of which were high in the differential. In this case muscle biopsy, following FDG PET scan, revealed histology in keeping with the clinical diagnosis of granulomatous vasculitis due to sarcoidosis. This demonstrates the need for clinicians to have a high index of suspicion for sarcoid myopathy, if the broader clinical picture is suggestive, even in the absence of classic or hallmark disease such as hilar or parenchymal lung disease.

Historically, three patterns of sarcoid myopathy are recognised:

- Chronic: Insidious onset of often proximal symmetric myalgia and weakness of limbs with demonstrable myopathy on neurophysiology. Biopsy tends to have granuloma and inflammatory infiltration with perivascular inflammation, as demonstrated in this case.
- Nodular: Multiple intramuscular nodular lesions, often tender, with normal serum muscle enzyme levels.
- Acute: The least common presentation, with acute and rapid onset proximal weakness with myalgia and elevated serum muscle enzyme levels and granulomas on biopsy.[1]

Previous assessments of organ involvement in sarcoidosis suggested low incidence of muscle involvement (0.4%), but the advent of newer imaging modalities such as FDG PET has aided recognition of extrapulmonary disease, with one study demonstrating 11.9% of a patient cohort with persistent disabling symptoms of sarcoidosis (58% of whom reported disabling arthralgia and/or muscle pain) had muscular PET avidity.[2,3] Tiger man sign refers to the relatively specific intense linear uptake seen on FDG PET in some cases of sarcoid myopathy.[4]

Learning points

- Sarcoid myopathy should be included in the differential diagnosis of any patient with a clinical myopathy and systemic illness alongside the broader differentials of infection, paraneoplastic process and primary systemic vasculitis.
- Pattern recognition of the clinical syndrome of sarcoidosis is essential in any atypical initial presentation of the disease and this usually includes one or more of the following: pulmonary involvement, hypercalcaemia,

hepatosplenomegaly, lymphadenopathy, ocular disease and cutaneous disease.

- Biopsy-proven granulomatous inflammation is essential in making the diagnosis and excluding alternative causes of myopathy.
- Normal creatine kinase and EMG studies may not exclude sarcoid myopathy.

Further reading

1. Bechman K., Christidis D., Walsh S., Birring S., and Galloway J., 2017. A review of the musculoskeletal manifestations of sarcoidosis. *Rheumatology,* 57(5), 777–783.
2. Baughman R., Teirstein A., Judson M., Rossman M. et al., 2001. Clinical characteristics of patients in a case-control study of sarcoidosis. *American Journal of Respiratory and Critical Care Medicine,* 164(1), 1885–1889.
3. Cremers J., Van Kroonenburgh M., Mostard R., Voo S. et al., 2014. Extent of disease activity assessed by 18F-FDG PET/CT in a Dutch sarcoidosis population. *Sarcoidosis Vasculitis and Diffuse Lung Diseases,* 18;31(1), 37–45.
4. Weers G., Lhommel R., Lecouvet F., Van Den Bergh P. and Lambert M., 2012. A tiger man. *The Lancet,* 380(9856), 1859.

CASE 23

Stefen Brady

History

A 70-year-old woman reported a 9-month history of myalgia and difficulty climbing the stairs. Six years earlier, she had developed similar symptoms which, at the time, were associated with an increased creatine kinase (CK) level of 8000 IU/L (normal = 25–200 IU/L).

On the previous presentation, her symptoms developed 12 months after she started taking a statin for hypercholesterolaemia. The statin was promptly withdrawn, and she was treated with high-dose prednisolone. She was back to her baseline within 6 to 12 months of starting treatment. The dose of prednisolone was then tapered over a further 6 months and discontinued.

Currently, she did not report any systemic symptoms and was not taking a statin or other treatment for hypercholesterolaemia. She had no family history of note.

Examination

There was bilateral, symmetrical, moderate hip flexion weakness (3/5) and mild shoulder abduction weakness (4/5) were identified.

Investigations

Her CK level was 5034 U/L (normal 25–200 U/L). A myositis immunoblot was positive for antibodies to 3-hydroxy-3-methyl-glutaryl-coenzyme A reductase (HMGCR). A muscle biopsy was performed and revealed minimal inflammation but for a few macrophages within scattered necrotic muscle fibres (Figure C23.1A). Immunostaining showed sarcolemmal labelling of scattered fibres with membrane attack complex (MAC or C5b-9) (Figure C23.1B), diffuse sarcoplasmic staining for p62 in several structurally normal muscle fibres (Figure C23.1C) and generalised mild upregulation of the inflammatory marker major histocompatibility complex (MHC) class I (Figure C23.1D). A PET-CT did not show changes suggestive of a malignancy.

Outcome

The patient was treated with high-dose oral glucocorticoids and methotrexate and made a complete recovery over the following 12–18 months. She remains on long-term methotrexate.

DOI: 10.1201/9780429429323-34

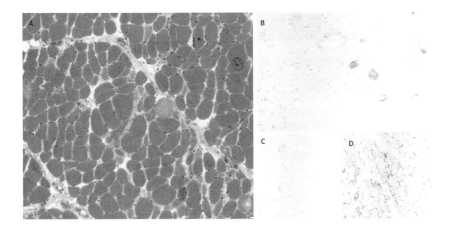

Figure C23.1 (A) Haematoxylin and eosin stain demonstrating myopathic muscle with frequent necrotic muscle fibres randomly scattered through fascicles (10×). Minimal inflammation observed in the perimysium (not shown). (B) Membrane attack complex (MAC or C5b-9) immunohistochemical (IHC) stain demonstrating cytoplasmic staining of necrotic fibres with focal sarcolemmal and capillary staining (20×). (C) p62 IHC stain showing a fine granular sarcoplasmic pattern of staining in necrotic fibres (20×). (D) Major histocompatibility complex (MHC) class 1 IHC stain demonstrating diffuse upregulation of sarcolemmal expression (10×).

DIAGNOSIS

Immune-mediated necrotising myopathy (IMNM) with antibodies to HMGCR.

Discussion

Statins are the most prescribed medication in the world and although they are well tolerated, they are not free from risk, being associated with three muscle syndromes or statin-related myopathies. In order of decreasing incidence, these conditions comprise myalgia with or without hyperCKaemia, rhabdomyolysis and immune-mediated necrotising myopathy (IMNM) (1).

Myalgia associated with statins usually affects the proximal lower limb muscles and may be exacerbated by exertion. There is no accompanying weakness. CK can be raised but is often normal. The clinical symptoms and serological abnormalities respond promptly and completely to statin withdrawal. If, in such a situation, a statin is believed to be highly beneficial, prescribing options to minimise symptoms include dose reduction or switching one statin for another, or using an alternative cholesterol lowering agent.

Rhabdomyolysis associated with statins is usually, if not always, iatrogenic. It is often the result of exposure to a large statin dose either by starting a high dose or suddenly increasing the dose following a cerebrovascular or cardiovascular event. It may also occur following the introduction of another medication that impairs statin metabolism. Common culprits for the latter include cardiovascular medications such as amiodarone or verapamil, and some antimicrobial medications, particularly erythromycin. The typical presentation of statin-related rhabdomyolysis is with myalgia, proximal weakness and myoglobinuria. The symptoms are usually widespread but may also be localised to certain muscle groups. Management again involves stopping the statin and any other offending medication combined with the institution of standard care for rhabdomyolysis such as intravenous fluid therapy to maintain adequate diuresis and monitoring for complications such as electrolyte and acid/base disturbance, compartment syndrome, renal failure and cardiac dysrhythmias. Some individuals may require analgesia.

IMNM is the term given to a group of muscle disorders grouped by similar pathological findings. Cases are associated with antibodies to HMGCR, the enzymatic target of statins, or signal recognition protein (SRP). A third group are seronegative IMNM, in which neither HMGCR nor SRP antibodies are present. HMGCR antibody-positive IMNM secondary to statins was first reported in 2010 (2).

Individuals with IMNM present with subacute, symmetric, proximal weakness without systemic symptoms. The CK level is typically markedly raised, often reaching levels of >5000 IU/L. In contrast, lower CK levels are typically observed in classic dermatomyositis associated with other autoantibodies. Muscle biopsy in IMNM reveals evidence of muscle fibre necrosis distributed randomly throughout the muscle with little associated inflammatory infiltrate. MHC class 1 staining confirms the inflammatory nature of the process but is often variably increased. MAC deposition on the sarcolemma of non-necrotic fibres is noted in up to 50% of cases. However, the most useful finding reported is the characteristic diffuse sarcoplasmic deposition of p62 in scattered muscle fibres (3).

Despite its strong association with statin usage, HMGCR antibody-positive IMNM is also reported in statin-naive individuals such as children and uncommonly in association with underlying malignancy in adults (4). It is therefore important to screen statin naïve antibody-positive adults for concomitant cancer.

The natural history of HMGCR-positive IMNM is uncertain (5). In most cases, the disease course is one of progressive weakness requiring aggressive immunotherapy. Initial treatment is with high-dose glucocorticoids often combined with a steroid-sparing agent such as methotrexate. Sometimes, those affected may require intravenous immunoglobulin and/or rituximab to help control the disease. Relapse many years after successful treatment is observed and, in these cases, it is appropriate to screen for malignancy even if the previous episode was associated with statin use. Early relapse is often due to inadequate glucocorticoid dosage and/or duration of treatment. Very few individuals will improve on withdrawal of the statin alone.

Learning points

- Statins are associated with three muscle-related presentations: myalgia with/without raised CK, rhabdomyolysis and HMGCR-positive immune-mediated necrotising myopathy (IMNM).
- IMNM is characterised by subacute, progressive, proximal weakness in the absence of marked systemic symptoms and accompanied by significantly raised CK levels.
- Muscle biopsy in IMNM shows prominent muscle fibre necrosis with minimal inflammation combined with characteristic p62 deposition in scattered muscle fibres.
- The natural history of statin-related HMGCR antibody-positive IMNM is uncertain and individuals usually require aggressive immunosuppressive therapy.
- HMGCR-positive IMNM is reported in association with cancer and therefore screening for malignant disease is appropriate in the absence of statins use.

Further reading

1. Hilton-Jones D. Statin-related myopathies. *Pract Neurol* 2018;18:97–105.
2. Christopher-Stine L, Casciola-Rosen LA, Hong G, et al. A novel autoantibody recognizing 200-kd and 100-kd proteins is associated with an immune-mediated necrotizing myopathy. *Arthritis Rheum* 2010;62:2757–66.
3. Norina Fischer, Corinna Preuße, Josefine Radke, et al. Sequestosome-1 (p62) expression reveals chaperone-assisted selective autophagy in immune-mediated necrotizing myopathies. *Brain Pathol.* 2020;30:261–71.

4. Allenbach Y, Keraen J, Bouvier AM, et al. High risk of cancer in autoimmune necrotizing myopathies: usefulness of myositis specific antibody. *Brain* 2016;139:2131–5.
5. Kushan Karunaratne, Dimitri Amiras, Matthew Pickering, et al. Autoimmune necrotising myopathy and HMGCR antibodies. *Pract Neurol* 2018;18:151–55.

CASE 24

Andria Merrison

PATIENT ASSESSMENT

History

A 24-year-old man was assaulted with a baseball bat and was found to have a large subdural haematoma on a CT scan of the head. His initial Glasgow Coma Scale (GCS) score was 13, but his score fluctuated within the first 48 hours of admission as a consequence of increasing problems with frontal contusions. He was transferred to the intensive care unit (ICU) following insertion of an intracranial pressure monitor and an extraventricular drain. His intracranial pressure was difficult to control and neuromuscular blockers were used as part of his management. He was also treated for a lower respiratory tract infection. He was ventilated for 28 days, requiring time to wean from ventilation.

Examination

During the course of his admission, this man developed weakness in all four limbs with reduced tone and mildly depressed reflexes.

Investigations

Creatine kinase (CK) was 1200. Nerve conduction studies and electromyography revealed an axonal sensorimotor neuropathy and a myopathy. A routine blood test screen for causes of neuropathy and myopathy was negative.

He made a good recovery over 6 months but continued to have mild bilateral foot drop and some sensory impairment in his feet.

DOI: 10.1201/9780429429323-35

DIAGNOSIS

Critical illness neuromyopathy.

Discussion

Patients requiring ICU support may acquire weakness due to critical illness polyneuropathy (CIP), critical illness myopathy (CIM) and/or muscle disuse atrophy. This may only become apparent when sedation is reduced and may manifest as difficulty weaning from ventilatory support. One-third of patients ventilated for >7 days have neuromuscular injury, 60–70% of those with sepsis/systemic inflammatory response syndrome (SIRS) or acute respiratory distress syndrome (ARDS), and 100% of those surviving septic shock and multi-organ failure (MOF).

CIP and CIM usually coexist and are associated with the same risk factors. These include prolonged ventilation, sepsis, ARDS, MOF, use of corticosteroids or neuromuscular blocking agents, poor glycaemic control and prolonged immobility. Propofol and benzodiazepines (used as sedatives in ICU) directly inhibit muscle excitability, worsening the effects of bed rest. Barbiturates and ketamine interact with N-methyl-D-aspartate receptors, which have an important role in muscle tropism.

Often CIM may predominate. Patients most commonly present with symmetric, flaccid weakness (often with depressed reflexes) with sparing of facial muscles. Whilst the diaphragm is often involved, diaphragmatic weakness is twice as common as neuromyopathy in the limbs – these two complications of critical illness may not correlate.

Muscle strength can be assessed by neurological examination and by using a grip myometer. CK levels can rise with necrosis/inflammation but may be normal. The diagnosis can be established by nerve conduction studies and electromyography. The neuropathy is axonal and usually involves both motor and sensory nerves.

Neurophysiological features include:

- Reduced amplitude compound muscle action potentials
- Increased muscle action potential duration
- Reduced amplitude sensory action potentials
- Normal: conduction velocities, distal motor latencies, response to repetitive nerve stimulation
- Fibrillation potentials and positive sharp waves may be seen 2–3 weeks into the course of the condition

Muscle biopsy is rarely needed in this context, but three main types of CIM are recognised: diffuse non-necrotising myopathy selective type 2 fibre atrophy, acute myosin-loss myopathy (often associated with steroids and/or neuromuscular blockers) and acute necrotising myopathy. Central nervous system causes of weakness should be excluded and pre-existing causes of weakness that may be unmasked by the physiological pressures of being critically ill.

Ways to prevent CIP/CIM are unclear. Optimising nutrition and minimising risk factors where possible may aid recovery. The role of early mobilisation is not yet established. Critical illness neuromyopathy is associated with prolonged hospital admissions and both increased long-term morbidity and mortality. Fifty per cent make a good long-term recovery but 25% may have significant long-term disability.

Learning points

- Critical illness neuromyopathy (neuropathy, myopathy and disuse atrophy) is the commonest cause of neuromuscular impairment in critically ill patients.
- Neuropathy and myopathy usually coexist but myopathy often predominates.
- Diaphragmatic weakness can occur in association with this condition, making weaning from ventilation challenging.
- A number of risk factors, including prolonged ventilation and sepsis, have been identified but ways to prevent it are unclear.
- Fifty per cent of patients make a good recovery but 25% are left with significant long-term disability.

Further reading

Boelens YFN, Melchers M & van Zanten ARH. 2022. Poor physical recovery after critical illness: incidence, features, risk factors, pathophysiology and evidence-based therapies. *Current Opinion Critical Care* 28(4): 409–416.

Griffiths RD & Hall JB. 2010. Intensive care unit-acquired weakness. *Critical Care Medicine* 38: 779–787.

Hermans G & Van den Burghe G. 2015. Clinical review: intensive care unit acquired weakness. *Critical Care* 19: 274.

Kelmenson DA, Held N, Allen RR, Quan D, Burnham EL, Clark BA, Ho PM, Kiser TH, Vandivier RW & Moss M. 2017. Outcomes of Intensive Care Unit patients with a discharge diagnosis of critical illness polyneuromyopathy: a propensity matched analysis. *Critical Care Medicine* 45(12): 2055–2060.

Kelmenson DA, Quan D & Moss M. 2018. What is the diagnostic accuracy of single nerve conduction studies and muscle ultrasound to identify critical illness polyneuropathy: a prospective cohort study. *Critical Care* 22(1): 342.

Klawitter F, Ehler J, Bajorat R & Patejdl R. 2023. Mitochondrial dysfunction in intensive care unit-acquired weakness and critical illness myopathy: a narrative review. *Int J Mol Sci* 24(6): 5516.

Lad H, Saumar TM, Herridge MS, Dos Santos CC, Mathur S, Batt J & Gilbert PM. 2020. Intensive care unit-acquired weakness: not just another muscle atrophying condition. *Int J Mol Sci* 21(21): 7840.

Muscle diseases

Piva S, Fagoni N & Latronico N. 2019. Intensive care unit-acquired weakness: unanswered questions and targets for future research. F1000 Research (open access) *Faculty Rev* 508. doi: 10.12688/f1000research.17376.

Vanhorebeek I Latronico N & Van den Berghe G. 2020. ICU-acquired weakness. *Intensive Care Medicine* 46(4): 637–653.

Younger DS. 2023. Critical illness-associated weakness and related motor disorders. *Handbook Clinical Neurology* 195: 707–777.

CASE 25

Louisa Kent and Stefen Brady

PATIENT ASSESSMENT

History

A 55-year-old woman presented with a 6-month history of progressive difficulty getting up from chairs and walking up stairs. On direct questioning, she reported difficulty hanging up her washing and changing the bedsheets. She also described increased fatigue and had stopped doing her usual hobbies after work. She had been commenced on a statin for hyperlipidaemia 12 months previously, but this had been stopped a month prior to her appointment after testing showed abnormal liver function.

Examination

She was overweight and had puffy facies, proximal upper and lower limb weakness, and a myopathic gait (also known as waddling or Trendelenburg gait). Her limb reflexes were unremarkable, although her ankle reflexes were slow to relax and there was myoedema on percussion of the quadriceps muscles.

Investigations

Her creatine kinase (CK) level was 800 IU/L (20–200 U/L). Repeat liver function tests demonstrated alanine aminotransferase (ALT) and aspartate aminotransferase (AST) levels just above the normal range. Her blood cholesterol was mildly raised.

DOI: 10.1201/9780429429323-36

DIAGNOSIS

Her thyroid-stimulating hormone (TSH) level was markedly raised, confirming a diagnosis of hypothyroid myopathy. Treatment with levothyroxine resulted in clinical improvement and normalisation of her biochemical abnormalities.

Discussion

Thyroid hormone disturbance is common and is also a well-recognised but sometimes overlooked, reversible cause of myopathy. Hypothyroidism can cause muscle symptoms including myalgia, stiffness and weakness. Examination findings are those classically seen in hypothyroidism and can include myxoedematous facies, dry skin, hair loss and slow pulse rate. Neuromuscular symptoms of hypothyroidism often comprise generalised slowness of movement, bilateral calf muscle hypertrophy and proximal weakness. Delayed and slow relaxation of tendon reflexes may be present (pseudomyotonia or "Woltman sign") and most easily noted with the ankle jerk reflex. Occasionally myoedema, or the "mounding phenomenon", is seen when direct percussion of the muscle elicits transient localised bulging of the muscle (see Further reading). However, the symptoms and signs of hypothyroidism can be subtle and can go unrecognised unless the condition is specifically considered.

CK in hypothyroid myopathy can range from normal to markedly elevated. Other investigation findings include anaemia, elevated liver enzymes (which may be of muscle and/or liver origin), hyperlipidaemia and hyponatraemia. If performed, electromyography (EMG) will show myopathic changes and spontaneous activity. There are no specific changes within the muscle biopsy in hypothyroid myopathy. However, in most cases, following a comprehensive clinical assessment and easy access to a thyroid function test, neither neurophysiological assessment nor muscle biopsy should be necessary.

Given its prevalence in the population, hypothyroidism should be considered in any patient presenting with proximal weakness before more esoteric diagnoses such as myositis or muscular dystrophy are considered. As with other endocrinopathy-associated myopathies, treatment of the underlying condition usually results in resolution of symptoms and signs. However, this may take some time.

In contrast to hypothyroidism, hyperthyroidism is a much less common cause of myopathy. These patients may also present with limb weakness and occasionally bulbar or respiratory muscle weakness. Examination findings include proximal muscle wasting and weakness, brisk reflexes and fasciculations mimicking amyotrophic lateral sclerosis. Systemic signs of thyrotoxicosis (weight loss, tremor, tachycardia and lid lag) or Graves' disease (exophthalmos, ophthalmoplegia, goitre, thyroid acropachy, and pretibial myxoedema) are typically observed following careful clinical examination. CK levels are usually normal in hyperthyroidism. EMG, if performed, may show myopathic features. A form of periodic paralysis can be caused by thyrotoxicosis. It is most common in Asian men, and typically manifests as proximal weakness which may develop following exercise, cold exposure or a meal high in carbohydrates, and can last hours to days. Thyrotoxicosis has also rarely been reported to cause rhabdomyolysis.

As thyroid disease can mimic a range of inherited and sporadic myopathies, it is important to ask about symptoms and look for signs of thyroid disease. It is strongly advised to check the TSH in every patient with symptoms and signs of muscle disease, or an unexplained deterioration in a patient known to have a myopathy, before embarking on more invasive investigations.

Learning points

- It is advisable to check TSH levels for any individual with symptoms or signs of muscle disease.
- Clinical history and examination will usually reveal systemic features of thyroid disease, negating the need for additional, more invasive investigation.
- Thyroid disease can worsen a pre-existing (diagnosed or undiagnosed) muscle disorder. This should be considered if symptoms persist or worsen despite adequate treatment for thyroid myopathy.
- Conversely, if there is unexplained or rapid deterioration in a patient known to have a myopathy, then performance of a TSH level is warranted.

Further reading

Capistrano and Galdino, Teaching Video NeuroImages: Myoedema in hypo-thyroidism, *Neurology*, January 26, 2015, https://doi.org/10.1212/WNL .0000000000001195

Mistry, Wass and Turner, When to consider thyroid dysfunction in the neurology clinic, *Practical Neurology*. 2009 Jun;9(3):145–56. https://doi.org/10 .1136/jnnp.2008.167163

CASE 26

Stefen Brady

PATIENT ASSESSMENT

A 17-year-old woman had been thoroughly investigated for raised serum trans-aminase levels, which had been identified on routine blood tests for fatigue. She had undergone a serological hepatitis screen, liver ultrasound and liver biopsy. At the conclusion of these examinations, she was additionally found to have a creatine kinase (CK) of 3500 IU/L (normal 25–200 U/L).

On further questioning, she did not report any symptoms suggestive of a myopathy. She enjoyed sports and played netball regularly at school and for her county team. She had never suffered from exercise-induced myalgia, contractures or myoglobinuria.

She had an older brother and sister, both of whom were healthy. A three-generation family pedigree was unremarkable and did not reveal any consanguinity. Her birth history and subsequent development were uneventful.

She had no other medical conditions and did not take any regular medications.

Examination
General and neurological examinations were normal.

Investigations
A repeat CK level showed continued elevation, at a level of 2900 U/L (normal 25–200 U/L). Initial genetic investigation for *DMD* deletions and duplications was negative.

DOI: 10.1201/9780429429323-37

DIAGNOSIS

ANO5-related hyperCKaemia.

Discussion

This case raises two separate important points. First, raised serum transaminases are not always indicative of liver disease and may originate from an unrecognised muscle disease. Second, when should and how best to investigate asymptomatic hyperCKaemia.

There are many causes for increased serum transaminase levels and often the reason for the elevation is clear. However, it is often forgotten that transaminases are present in muscle. As a result, it is not unusual to see cases, such as the one described here, where a patient with asymptomatic or paucisymptomatic hyper-CKaemia has undergone extensive, costly and sometimes potentially hazardous investigations before creatine kinase (CK) levels are checked. Both alanine aminotransferase (ALT) and aspartate aminotransferase (AST) are present in muscle. A clue as to the origin of raised transaminases is the serum gamma-glutamyl transferase (γGT or GGT), which is not present in muscle and is therefore not elevated in muscle-related transaminase elevation.

How to define and best investigate asymptomatic hyperCKaemia is uncertain and thus there are several guidelines and algorithms which can be followed (1–3). There are two factors which render decision-making difficult in investigation of hyperCKemia. The first is that many normal people's CK levels fall outside the quoted upper limit of normal and therefore do not reflect a pathogenic finding.

What is a normal CK depends on several factors, particularly race, sex, age, and the level and type of physical exercise undertaken by the individual (4, 5). CK levels are generally higher in Afro-Caribbean individuals compared to Caucasians, in men compared to women and in the young in contrast to the old. There is guidance on modifying the CK range to consider the effects of race and sex (6). Most physical exercise does not have a profound impact on the CK. Having said that, individuals who regularly participate in very physical or prolonged exercise can routinely have CKs in the thousands. These activities include bodybuilding, weightlifting and marathon running. A simple method for confirming whether a raised CK is related to exertion, is to recheck it after the individual has refrained from strenuous physical exertion for 7 days. In most cases, the CK will return to normal or near normal and no further investigation is required.

The second confounding factor is the presence of three CK isoenzymes in serum (CK-MM, CK-MB and CK-BB) which are predominantly found in skeletal muscle, cardiac muscle and brain tissue, respectively. Thus, the causes of raised CK are varied and not always indicative of a myopathy.

If an elevated CK cannot be explained by race or sex, or persists despite temporary cessation of physical exercise, or is just too high to ignore (rule of thumb >1000 IU/L), there are several causes to be considered. It is helpful to categorise them into (1) uncommon primary myopathies and (2) common miscellaneous causes. The underlying causes in this latter category of asymptomatic or paucisymptomatic hyperCKaemia include medications (most commonly statins especially if combined with a medication that inhibits statin metabolism), endocrinopathies (most commonly hypothyroidism) and recreational drug use.

Although uncommon, significantly raised CKs, as high as 2000 U/L, can be observed in cases of denervation. A cause of hyperCKaemia that is often not considered or considered only after more expensive tests have been performed is macroCK. Two types of macroCK – type I and type II – are described. The cause of both is an increase in the half-life of CK. In type I, CK is complexed to immunoglobulin. In type II, oligomeric mitochondrial CK is present in serum. MacroCK is observed in inflammatory and neoplastic diseases and can be detected by electrophoresis.

Primary myopathic, asymptomatic or paucisymptomatic, causes of raised CK are rare. Causative genes include *DMD* in women and the limb girdle muscular dystrophy genes in women and men: *CAV3, CAPN, DYSF, FKRP* and *ANO5*. Some individuals will go on to develop weakness later in life, and cardiac screening is important for those known to carry pathogenic variants in genes associated with cardiac diseases such as *DMD*. Other causes which should be considered are early Pompe disease, which may be accompanied by minimal symptoms and signs, amyopathic connective tissue disease or the early stage of an inflammatory myopathy.

Learning points

- A raised CK is common and often not associated with a primary myopathy.
- The quoted normal range for CK is conservative and an individual's race, sex, age and participation in strenuous activity should be considered when deciding on the need for further investigation.
- In those individuals with a moderately raised, asymptomatic hyperCKaemia (<1000 IU/L in Caucasian men and <1500 IU/L in Afro-Caribbean men) without obvious cause, combined with a normal examination, normal investigations for thyroid disease and an unremarkable neurophysiological assessment, further investigation is unlikely to bear fruit.

Further reading

1. Kim EJ, Wierzbicki AS. Investigating raised creatine kinase. *BMJ*. 2021 Jun 23;373:n1486. doi: 10.1136/bmj.n1486. PMID: 34162592.
2. Silvestri NJ, Wolfe GI. Asymptomatic/pauci-symptomatic creatine kinase elevations (hyperckemia). *Muscle Nerve*. 2013 Jun;47(6):805–815. doi: 10.1002/mus.23755. Epub 2013 Apr 29. PMID: 23625835.
3. Kyriakides T, Angelini C, Schaefer J, Sacconi S, Siciliano G, Vilchez JJ and Hilton-Jones D. (2010), EFNS guidelines on the diagnostic approach to pauci- or asymptomatic hyperCKemia. *European Journal of Neurology*. 2010; 17: 767–773.

4. Neal RC, Ferdinand KC, Ycas J, Miller E. Relationship of ethnic origin, gender, and age to blood creatine kinase levels. *The American Journal of Medicine.* 2009 Jan;122(1):73–78. doi: 10.1016/j.amjmed.2008.08.033. PMID: 19114174.

5. Bekkelund SI. Leisure physical exercise and creatine kinase activity. The Tromsø study. *Scandinavian Journal of Medicine & Science in Sports.* 2020 Dec;30(12):2437–2444. doi: 10.1111/sms.13809. Epub 2020 Sep 18. PMID: 32799358.

6. Moghadam-Kia S, Oddis CV, Aggarwal R. Approach to asymptomatic creatine kinase elevation. *Cleveland Clinic Journal of Medicine.* 2016 Jan;83(1):37-42. doi: 10.3949/ccjm.83a.14120. PMID: 26760521; PMCID: PMC4871266.

CASE 27

Stefen Brady

History

A fit and healthy 72-year-old man was referred for assessment. He had first been seen 2 years earlier in the movement disorders clinic and diagnosed with early Parkinson disease complicated by head drop. A whole-spine MRI was unremarkable and did not reveal an alternative structural cause for the head drop. An initial trial of Levodopa treatment was ineffective.

On review in the neuromuscular clinic, the patient recalled pain in his neck and shoulders when riding his motorcycle beginning 6 years prior to presentation. As time progressed, he found that he was unable to hold his head up when wearing his motorcycle helmet. He continued to ride a bicycle daily but had increasing difficulty controlling his head. More recently, he had noticed that he needed to support his head on his hands when sitting and watching television or when talking with friends.

He denied the presence of weakness beyond his head and neck and did not complain of any of the motor or non-motor symptoms typically associated with Parkinson disease. He was one of nine siblings and had no family history of note.

Examination

The main finding on neurological examination was the identification of thinning of the neck extensor muscles and marked weakness (MRC grade 2) of neck extension.

Investigations

His creatine kinase (CK) level was 126 U/L (normal 25–200 U/L) and a dried blood spot for alpha-glucosidase activity was normal (excluding Pompe disease). Nerve conduction studies were normal, however, electromyography (EMG) showed widespread myopathic changes in the paraspinal muscles. Review of the initial whole-spine MRI performed 2 years earlier revealed diffuse fatty atrophy of the paraspinal muscles (Figure C27.1).

DOI: 10.1201/9780429429323-38

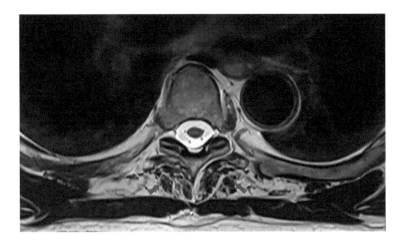

Figure C27.1 T1-weighted axial MRI sections through the spine showing fatty atrophy of the paraspinal muscles, which can be easily missed when not specifically sought.

DIAGNOSIS

Isolated neck extensor myopathy (axial myopathy).

Discussion

Isolated neck extensor myopathy (INEM) is a neuromuscular disorder affecting older patients. As with many myopathies, disease progression is gradual over many years. The initial complaint is often neck or shoulder pain followed by progressive weakness of neck extension resulting in head drop. As the condition progresses, those affected struggle to walk as they cannot see ahead and will adopt a recumbent position or support their head with a hand under the chin when sitting. Eating can be challenging and travelling by motor vehicle is particularly problematic, as those affected lack the necessary strength to control their head as the car accelerates or brakes. This is often worse when they travel as passengers and during emergency braking. Despite these problems, those affected often cope well.

The differential diagnosis of head drop is wide and includes myopathic and non-myopathic neurological disorders such as motor neurone disease (MND), myasthenia gravis (MG) and Parkinson disease (PD). The non-myopathic causes are significantly more common in the population and should always be considered first. Therefore, symptoms and signs of MND, MG and PD, such as upper motor neurone signs, fatigability, fasciculations, bradykinesia and the non-motor features of PD, should be carefully sought.

As emphasised in a recent review, axial weakness is a feature of many muscle diseases (1). In muscle clinics, it is most often observed in patients with myotonic dystrophy type 1, but it is also described in sporadic muscle disease (e.g., inclusion body myositis [IBM]), muscular dystrophies congenital myopathies (e.g., *RYR1*-related myopathy) and metabolic myopathies (e.g., Pompe disease). However, in the absence of additional symptoms and signs beyond the weakness of neck extension and minimal limb girdle weakness, the diagnosis will invariably be isolated neck extensor myopathy. Features such as cramps and myoglobinuria, non-positional dysphagia, contractures, respiratory failure or marked weakness beyond the axial muscles should prompt consideration of alternative diagnoses.

Excluding MRI, investigations can be unremarkable in INEM, with their main use being to exclude alternative diagnoses. In INEM, CK is usually within the normal range. EMG is the most useful investigation in excluding alternative diagnosis, by helping to identify neurogenic changes and impaired neuromuscular transmission associated with MND and MG, respectively. The presence of myotonia in the paraspinal muscles is suggestive but not diagnostic of the metabolic myopathy, Pompe disease. Extensive myopathic change on EMG beyond the paraspinal muscles would argue against a diagnosis of INEM.

Management of INEM follows a supportive path. Those affected can largely be reassured that INEM is a slowly progressive sporadic disorder limited to the axial muscles. Cervical collars may help irrespective of the underlying diagnosis of head drop and should be used when those affected travel by motorised transport, such as car, coach or train. In rare cases, spinal fusion is considered and can be highly effective (2) but also quite limiting.

Learning points

- Head drop is observed in several myopathic and non-myopathic neurological diseases.
- The most common causes are non-myopathic and include motor neurone disease, myasthenia gravis and Parkinson disease.
- INEM is the likely diagnosis in an elderly individual with head drop in the absence of additional symptoms and signs.
- Investigations should include CK, EMG and spinal MRI. Paraspinal muscle biopsy is not recommended because of the frequent presence of non-specific findings.
- Cervical collars are helpful and spinal surgery will have a role in a small number of cases.

Further reading

1. Witting N, Andersen LK, Vissing J. Axial myopathy: an overlooked feature of muscle diseases. *Brain* 2016;139:13–22.
2. Karunaratne K, Wade C, Lehovsky J, Viegas S. Spinal surgery for a late-onset axial myopathy. *BMJ Case Rep.* 2021;14:e240738.

CASE 28

Stefen Brady

PATIENT ASSESSMENT

History

An 18-year-old woman was referred to the neuromuscular clinic with a history of exercise intolerance and myalgia. Her symptoms always started within the first few minutes of exercising. She could neither sprint nor walk up an incline without stopping, but she could play a whole game of hockey without difficulty after gently warming up. Her symptoms had affected her for as long as she could remember. She had no weakness and did not report exertional muscle contractures. She had not experienced any episodes of myoglobinuria (black tea- or cola-coloured urine). She had no family history of note.

Examination

Neurological examination was unremarkable but for the presence of mild asymmetric scapular winging.

Investigations

An elevated resting creatine kinase (CK) of 6771 IU/L (normal 40–320 IU/L) was observed following testing in clinic. A non-ischaemic forearm exercise test revealed a rise in serum ammonia (ΔNH_3, 162 µmol/L) but no increase in serum lactate. A muscle biopsy showed mild variation in muscle fibre diameters with subsarcolemmal and sarcoplasmic vacuoles (Figure C28.1A). The vacuoles contained glycogen on periodic acid-Schiff (PAS) staining (Figure C28.1B). There was a complete absence of myophosphorylase staining (Figure C28.1C and D).

DOI: 10.1201/9780429429323-39

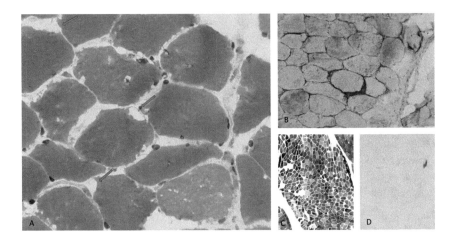

Figure C28.1 A. Haematoxylin and eosin stain demonstrating the presence of variably sized subsarcolemmal vacuoles (blue arrows) (20x). (B) Periodic acid-Schiff (PAS) histochemical (HC) stain highlighting glycogen accumulation in the subsarcolemmal vacuoles (20x). (C) Normal control myophosphorylase HC stain demonstrating diffuse "blue" positive staining. (D) Myophosphorylase HC stain revealing the complete absence of myophosphorylase activity in McArdle disease.

DIAGNOSIS

Glycogen storage disorder (GSD) V (McArdle disease) due to compound hetero-zygous mutations in *PYGM*.

Discussion

McArdle disease is the commonest of the glycogen storage disorders. It is the result of biallelic pathogenic variants in the *PYGM* gene, which encodes muscle protein glycogen phosphorylase (myophosphorylase) catalysing the first step in muscle glycolysis. The accepted prevalence of this condition is 1:100,000, but it is believed that this may be an underestimate.

McArdle disease has a characteristic clinical presentation of myalgia and cramps occurring within the first few minutes of exercising or triggered by sustained isometric contraction. The second wind phenomenon is a clinical symptom that is pathognomonic of McArdle disease. It describes an improvement in the initial exertional symptoms after about 8–10 minutes of aerobic activity after which, the affected individual can continue exercising. This phenomenon is well recognised and reported by most patients and can be provoked and observed during exercise testing. The improvement in symptoms and exercise tolerance is believed to be due to the delivery of glucose from the liver and fatty acids to exercising muscles.

Other features observed in McArdle disease are muscle contracture during activity, rhabdomyolysis (50%), and, rarely, compartment syndrome or renal failure. A significant percentage of patients, usually those over 40 years of age, will develop fixed upper limb weakness. Atypical presentations of McArdle disease have been reported and range from axial myopathy to pauci- or asymptomatic hyperCK-aemia, and a facioscapulohumeral muscular dystrophy (FSHD)-like phenotype. Electrocardiogram (ECG) changes, cardiomyopathy, ischaemic heart disease and retinopathy are rarely reported in association with McArdle and are not frequent enough to support screening.

Of note, activities not commonly thought of as exercise such as chewing (1), sexual intercourse or emotionally intense situations (2), such as cheering at a sports match, can provoke myalgia, myoglobinuria, muscle contracture and even rhab-domyolysis in individuals with McArdle disease. The cause is likely to be sustained isometric muscle contraction.

Despite its characteristic presentation, 90% of individuals with McArdle disease initially receive an incorrect medical diagnosis. Frequently, childhood symptoms are attributed to "growing pains" (3), and a history of such symptoms should be viewed with suspicion. The delay to correct diagnosis is exemplified by the median onset of symptoms being 3 years of age and yet the median age of diagnosis is 33 years of age (3). Ancillary investigations are helpful. The CK level is elevated in nearly all patients and serum hyperuricaemia is common. A non-ischaemic fore-arm exercise test will reveal an excessive rise in ammonia and a blunted lactate response to exertion in patients with McArdle disease. If performed, a muscle biopsy will typically reveal subsarcolemmal vacuoles containing glycogen and absent myophosphorylase activity (Figure C28.1). In recent years, however, both the non-ischaemic forearm exercise test and muscle biopsy have been superseded by molecular genetic testing. Eighty-five per cent of UK and Northern European patients with McArdle disease harbour p.Arg50X and pGly205Ser pathogenic variants in *PYGM*. As a result, the first-line investigation is hotspot analysis by gene sequencing or now, more frequently, whole-genome sequencing.

Despite the onset of symptoms with exercise, aerobic exercise is safe and beneficial for patients with McArdle disease. In general, exercise involving isometric muscle contraction should be avoided (i.e., planks, leg lifts and wall sits). Advice on appropriate exercise regimens should be sought from a specialist neuromuscular centre.

Learning points

- McArdle disease is the commonest glycogen storage disorder (GSD) and it has a characteristic, arguably diagnostic, clinical presentation.
- The second wind phenomenon is pathognomonic and recognised by individuals with McArdle disease, but its significance is commonly missed by clinicians.
- Diagnostic testing should start with genetic testing, which may involve hotspot mutation testing of *PYGM* at some centres or a next-generation sequencing (NGS) panel at other centres (where available).
- Aerobic exercise is safe, but advice on physical activity should be sought from a specialist neuromuscular centre.

Further reading

1. Kouwenberg CV, Voermans NC, Quinlivan R, van den Engel-Hoek L. Mastication and oral motor function in McArdle disease: Patient reported complaints. *Journal of Neuromuscular Disorders*. 2018;5:353–357.
2. Brady S, Godfrey R, Scalco RS, *et al.* Emotionally-intense situations can result in rhabdomyolysis in McArdle disease. *BMJ Case Reports*. 2014;2014:bcr2013203272.
3. Renata Siciliani Scalco, Jasper M. Morrow, Suzanne Booth, *et al.* Misdiagnosis is an important factor for diagnostic delay in McArdle disease. *Neuromuscular Disorders*. 2017;27:852–855.

CASE 29

Andria Merrison

PATIENT ASSESSMENT

History

A 49-year-old woman presented with a 1–2-year history of mildly progressive weakness in the lower limbs. Rising from a seated position had become more difficult and she had found stairs to be more of a struggle with time. She reported generalised aches and pains, including low back pain, intermittently requiring analgesia. She also reported quite profound fatigue and a variable sleep pattern.

This woman had a longstanding history of anxiety and depression and had been taking antidepressants. She had two children who were well and did not report any family history of neuromuscular disease.

Examination

On examination, there was mild proximal weakness in the upper limbs, grade 4+/5 and moderate proximal weakness in the lower limbs grade 4/5. There was no focal wasting or fasciculation. Reflexes were present and symmetrical and plantars flexor All cranial nerves and all sensory modalities were intact.

Investigations

Creatine kinase (CK) was raised at 808 U/l. Plasma viscosity, thyroid function, antinuclear antibody and myositis antibody tests were normal or negative. Vitamin D levels were low at 38 and vitamin D supplementation was given.

Nerve conduction studies were normal. Electromyography (EMG) showed minor changes in the deltoid muscles only.

A muscle biopsy showed mild non-specific myopathic changes. There were no vacuoles and both glycogen and acid phosphatase activity levels appeared normal.

Forced vital capacity was 48% of predicted and overnight oximetry revealed significant dips in oxygenation. Non-invasive ventilation was initiated at night, which led to a markedly improved sleep pattern and some improvement in daytime fatigue levels.

A Pompe dry blood spot analysis was initially normal with acid alpha-glucosidase (GAA) levels of 8.45 pmol/punch/hour (normal >3.88 pmol/punch/hour). Repeat testing revealed a level of 4.5 pmol/punch/hour.

Genetic testing identified a mutation in the GAA gene on chromosome 17.

DOI: 10.1201/9780429429323-40

DIAGNOSIS

Acid maltase deficiency (Pompe disease or glycogen storage disorder II).

Discussion

Acid maltase deficiency (also known as Pompe disease or glycogen storage disorder II and a lysosomal storage disorder) is an autosomal recessive metabolic myopathy caused by mutations in the GAA gene on chromosome 17q25.3 encoding acid α-1,4-glucosidase (GAA) or acid maltase. It was first described in 1932 and since then over 600 different mutations have been reported.

Acid maltase or GAA is a lysosomal enzyme involved in the conversion of glycogen to glucose. Deficiency leads to accumulation of glycogen in lysosomes of several different tissues including cardiac, skeletal and smooth muscle cells. Vasculopathy and cognitive impairment can form part of this condition. Pathogenesis may be directly due to the accumulation of glycogen causing displacement of cellular organelles, abnormal lysosomal activity promoting autophagy and other effects on intermediary metabolism.

The most common form is adult onset with slowly progressive symmetrical proximal limb (often lower limb predominant) and respiratory muscle weakness. In one-third of adult cases, respiratory complications (due to respiratory muscle or isolated diaphragmatic weakness) are the presenting feature. Respiratory problems also arise due to disruption of proximal and distal airway structure. Some patients develop spine rigidity, scoliosis, ptosis and/or swallowing problems. In those presenting in adulthood, there is usually some residual GAA activity of 10–30% of normal. Unlike other glycogenoses, hypoglycaemia does not occur in acid maltase deficiency. This condition is an important differential for muscular dystrophy, particularly limb girdle muscular dystrophy.

Two other phenotypes are recognised. First, there is a classic infantile form which leads to more severe proximal muscle weakness (due to GAA inactivity); enlargement of the tongue; feeding difficulties; and heart, liver and respiratory insufficiency. Untreated, most patients die before the age of 3 years. There is also a non-classic infantile form which is milder and usually presents in the first years of life. In this form, respiratory and skeletal muscles are affected but cardiac involvement is rare.

GAA levels can be measured in blood (dry bloodspot) and analysis of lymphocytes shows evidence of glycogen granules. Dry bloodspot analysis is used in some countries for newborn screening.

In contrast to infantile forms where histological features are usually diagnostic, in adult cases a muscle biopsy may not always exhibit the expected changes. Characteristic muscle biopsy features of Pompe disease include sarcoplasmic vacuoles within myofibres visible on routine H&E stains (Figure C29.1A). These vacuoles contain glycogen (as evidenced by periodic acid-Schiff staining) and increased acid phosphatase activity (Figure C29.1B and C). Electron microscopy

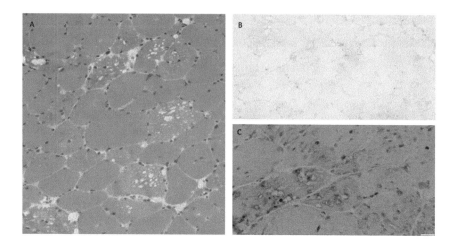

Figure C29.1 Pompe Disease. A. H&E 20× demonstrating multiple vacuoles within muscle fibres on background of myopathic changes. B. PAS 20× demonstrating increased glycogen content within vacuoles. C. Acid Phosphatase 20× highlighting increased activity within vacuoles due to increased lysosomal activity (red staining).

may be helpful in confirming the glycogen content of the vacuoles. Enzyme assays can also be performed on muscle, liver or skin fibroblasts. However, genetic analysis is the most reliable diagnostic modality and can be used to identify gene carriers.

Treatment involves intravenous replacement therapy with recombinant α-glucosidase (Myozyme), which has been available since 2006. This has a major impact on survival and cardiomyopathy in infantile Pompe disease, with some patients now surviving into adulthood. The efficacy of therapy is more difficult to assess in adult-onset cases, but there is evidence that replacement therapy can improve mobility and stabilise respiratory function. Avalglucosidase alfa-ngpt (Nexviazyme), a synthetic oligosaccharide available since 2021, offers an alternative Pompe disease treatment and may be more effective in reducing the accumulation of glycogen. A number of gene-modifying avenues are being explored for Pompe disease, providing an attractive way of treating the multisystem complications, including central nervous system manifestations where conventional treatments are limited by the blood–brain barrier. This includes using recombinant adenovirus and lentivirus vectors.

People living with Pompe disease will also require lifelong multidisciplinary supportive therapy. This is likely to include respiratory and cardiac support. The first patients treated with enzyme replacement therapy in infancy are now surviving into adulthood with this multidisciplinary approach to care.

Learning points

- Acid maltase deficiency is a potentially treatable form of metabolic muscle disease. It is currently treated with enzyme replacement therapy and a number of gene-modifying therapeutic approaches are being trialled.
- This condition is frequently associated with respiratory failure, with respiratory compromise being the presenting feature in one-third of adult-onset cases.
- Cardiac involvement is common in the more severe classic infantile-onset cases but less likely in adult-onset cases. Cardiac outcomes are better in those receiving early initiation of enzyme replacement therapy.
- Unlike other glycogenoses, hypoglycaemia does not tend to occur.
- Diagnosis can be made by measuring GAA in blood, analysing glycogen granules in lymphocytes and genetic analysis.
- With treatment, patients with infantile-onset may survive into adulthood and those with adult-onset disease may experience improvements in mobility and stabilisation of respiratory function.

Further reading

Dangouloff T, Boemer F & Servais L. 2021. Newborn screening of neuromuscular disease. *Neuromuscular Disorders* 31(10): 1070–1080.

Dornelles AD, Junges APP, Pereira TV, Krug BC, Goncalves CBT, Llerena JC, Kishnani PS, de Oliveira HA & Schwartz IVD. 2021. A systematic review and meta-analysis of enzyme replacement therapy in late-onset Pompe disease. *Journal of Clinical Medicine* 10(21): 4828.

Iolascon G, Vitacca M, Carroro E, Chisari C, Fiore P, Messina S, Mongini TEG, Sansone VA, Toscano A & Siciliano G. 2018. The role of rehabilitation in the management of late-onset Pompe disease: a narrative review of the level of evidence. *Acta Myologica* 37(4): 241–251.

Leon-Astudillo C, Trivedi PD, Sun RC, Gentry MS, Fuller DD, Byrne BJ & Corti M. 2023. Current avenues of gene therapy in Pompe disease. *Current Opinion in Neurology* 36(5): 464–473.

Platt FM, d'Azzo A, Davidson BL, Neufeld EF & Tifft CJ. 2018. Lysosomal storage diseases. *Nature Reviews Disease Primers* 4(1): 27.

Sarah B, Giovanna B, Emanuela K, Nadi N, Jose V & Alberto P. 2022. Clinical efficacy of the enzyme replacement therapy in patients with late-onset Pompe disease: a systematic review and meta-analysis. *Journal of Neurology* 269(2): 733–741.

Schoser B & Laforet P. 2022. Therapeutic thoroughfares for adults living with Pompe disease. *Current Opinion in Neurology* 35(5): 645–650.

Shah NM, Sharma L, Ganeshamoorthy S & Kaltsakas G. 2020. Respiratory failure and sleep-disordered breathing in late-onset Pompe disease: a narrative review. *Thoracic Disease* 12(S2): S235–S247.

CASE 30

Stefen Brady

PATIENT ASSESSMENT

History

A 38-year-old man was reviewed in the neuromuscular clinic several months after being admitted to hospital with myalgia, proximal weakness and black tea-/cola-coloured urine. His creatine kinase (CK) on admission was 75,000 U/L (normal = 40–320 U/L). His symptoms commenced within hours of returning home following a transatlantic flight. His CK dramatically decreased over the course of a few days with intravenous fluid administration and he was discharged home within 7 days.

In clinic, he described feeling unwell towards the end of his trip with symptoms of a febrile coryzal illness. As a result, he had not eaten much prior to or during his flight home. Further questioning revealed that he had experienced multiple episodes of myalgia and myoglobinuria since adolescence. Some, but not all, occurred following prolonged exercise. The most memorable episode occurred during his honeymoon when he combined a strenuous cycling holiday with a not inconsiderable amount of wine. Despite his symptoms, he had always enjoyed exercise but had become more sedentary with age.

He did not take any regular medication. He had no family history of note.

Examination

Neurological and systemic examination were normal.

Investigations

His resting CK level was 278 IU/L (40–320 IU/L). Genetic testing established the diagnosis.

DOI: 10.1201/9780429429323-41

DIAGNOSIS

Fatty acid oxidation disorder (FAOD), carnitine palmitoyltransferase II (CPT II) deficiency.

Discussion

The symptoms in this case are those of rhabdomyolysis. Inherited causes of rhabdomyolysis are rare and genetically heterogeneous, comprising FAODs, as, in this case, glycogen storage disorders (GSDs), mitochondrial myopathy, congenital myopathy, and muscular dystrophy including Becker muscular dystrophy and limb girdle muscular dystrophy due to pathogenic variants in *CAV3*, *ANO5*, *FKRP* or *DYSF*. CPT II deficiency is due to compound heterozygous mutations in *CPT2*. CPT II is involved in, primarily, fatty acid (FA) β-oxidation and, along with other proteins, the transport of long-chain FAs across the mitochondrial membrane.

Commoner causes of rhabdomyolysis include recreational drug use, medications such as statins, especially if the dose is increased precipitously or statin metabolism is inhibited by the introduction of another medication, and unaccustomed exercise. The most important question for the clinician when a patient presents with rhabdomyolysis, after commencing appropriate treatment, is whether to investigate for an inherited cause. One helpful mnemonic which may help direct further investigations is RHABDO (Table C30.1) [1].

A careful clinical history can often differentiate between FAODs and GSDs. Glucose and glycogen are a muscle's primary energy source during the first minutes of exercise and during high-intensity exercise. With longer duration exercise (>30 minutes) and when fasting, there is an increasing reliance on FA β-oxidation. Thus, symptoms arising early, in the first minutes of exercise or with a sudden increase in exercise tempo are indicative of a GSD, whereas symptoms arising during or after prolonged exercise or fasting are suggestive of an FAOD. Febrile illness, extremes of ambient temperature, certain medications and general anaesthetic can also trigger rhabdomyolysis in those with a FAOD.

Table C30.1 When to further investigate an episode of rhabdomyolysis – RHABDO

Recurrent episodes of exertional rhabdomyolysis
HyperCKaemia more than 8 weeks after event
Accustomed to exercise
Blood creatine kinase (CK) concentration above 50× upper limit of normal
Drug ingestion insufficient to explain exertional rhabdomyolysis
Other family members affected or other exertional symptoms

Source: Fernandes PM, Davenport RJ, How to do it: investigate exertional rhabdomyolysis (or not), *Practical Neurology* 2019;19:43–48.

FAODs can present at any age. CPT II deficiency is clinically divided into three phenotypes: lethal neonatal form; severe infantile form; and mild adult form, which is characterised by episodic rhabdomyolysis presenting at almost any age between childhood and adulthood. The severe multisystem neonatal-/infantile-onset forms are typified by hypoketotic hypoglycaemia, weakness, hepatic failure and cardiomyopathy. In the adult form of CPT II deficiency, interictal CK is usually normal and the serum acylcarnitine profile shows an increase in long-chain FAs.

Investigation of rhabdomyolysis and metabolic myopathy has radically changed in recent years because of access to next-generation sequencing (NGS). It is now cost-effective to go straight to a gene panel. Prior to this, investigation could be a lengthy process including testing of any or all of the following: serum lactate, acylcarnitine profile, alpha-glucosidase activity, urinary organic acids, non-ischaemic forearm exercise testing, skin biopsy and fibroblast culture, muscle biopsy, (some of the histopathological features observed if a muscle biopsy is performed are shown in Figure C30.1), and finally sequential genetic testing of individual genes known to cause (at the time) rhabdomyolysis. Often the more invasive investigations are now used to assess the pathogenicity of variants of uncertain significance identified through NGS.

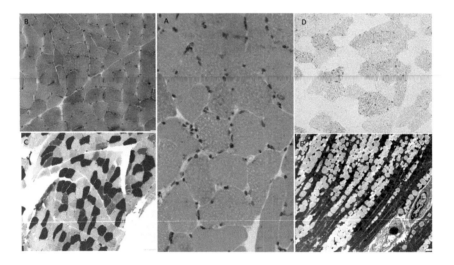

Figure C30.1 Lipid myopathy (fatty acid oxidation disorder). (A) Haematoxylin and eosin stain demonstrating mild myopathic variation in fibre size with numerous stippled fibres (10x). (B) Modified Gömöri trichrome stain confirming the presence of numerous unrimmed vacuoles within type 1 fibres (20x). (C) Metachromatic ATPase histochemical stain confirming the presence of vacuoles within type 1 (dark blue) muscle fibres (10x). (D) Oil Red O lipid stain revealing a marked increase in lipid storage within type 1 muscle fibres (20x). (E) Electron microscopy confirming a marked increase in lipids within muscle.

Management of FAODs is focused on patient education about:

1. Avoiding triggers
2. Appropriate exercise and dietary advice including avoidance of dieting and fasting, increased dietary slow-release carbohydrates, and reduction of fat
3. Recognition of the symptoms rhabdomyolysis and when to seek medical attention because of the risk of renal failure and hyperkalaemia and, infrequently, death

Learning points

- FAODs are a rare genetically heterogeneous group of autosomal recessive disorders that can present with rhabdomyolysis between childhood and adulthood. CPT II deficiency is one of the commoner FAODs and inherited causes of rhabdomyolysis.
- A careful history can differentiate FAODs and GSDs.
- Interictal CK is usually normal or mildly raised in FAOD.
- Management includes: the avoidance of triggers, advice on exercise and diet, and education on the recognition and treatment of rhabdomyolysis.

Further reading

1. Fernandes PM, Davenport RJ. How to do it: investigate exertional rhabdomyolysis (or not). *Practical Neurology* 2019;19:43–48.

CASE 31

Stefen Brady

Example 1

History

A 32-year-old man presented 4 days after the start of a cycling holiday with increasing proximal lower limb myalgia and stiffness. His creatine kinase (CK) was 47,000 U/L (normal = 40–320 U/L) and he was admitted to hospital for management of rhabdomyolysis.

He was a keen cyclist and reported similar but less severe symptoms with prolonged exercise throughout his life. There was no history of black tea- or cola-coloured urine following exercise. There was no additional significant past medical history or family history of note.

Examination following recovery revealed mild scoliosis, and finger flexion and Achilles contractures.

Example 2

History

A 56-year-old Caucasian man was referred after the discovery of an elevated serum CK level of 1250 U/L (normal = 40–320 U/L) following extensive investigation for elevated transaminase levels. He reported difficulty building muscle as a younger man but was otherwise asymptomatic. He did not enjoy sports and had not exercised for several decades. Family history revealed that an older brother had suffered an episode of malignant hyperthermia when having his tonsils removed in adolescence.

Examination
The muscles were well defined, mildly hypertrophied and there was no wasting. The neurological examination was otherwise normal.

Investigations
Serum CK was 1250U/L. Genetic testing established the diagnosis.

DOI: 10.1201/9780429429323-42

DIAGNOSIS

Autosomal dominant *RYR1*-related myopathy.

Discussion

RYR1 is a large 106 exon-long gene which encodes a calcium channel (RyR1) located in the sarcoplasmic reticulum (SR). RyR1 plays a vital role in muscle excitation-contraction coupling. Genetic defects in *RYR1* result in several muscle disorders which are genetically, phenotypically and histopathologically varied. Both autosomal recessive (AR) and autosomal dominant (AD) forms have been reported. AR *RYR1*-related disorders tend to be more clinically severe. Adult-onset RYR1-related disease is usually AD.

Clinical manifestations include scoliosis and joint contractures, malignant hyperthermia (MH), axial weakness, muscle hypertrophy and exercise-induced symptoms including rhabdomyolysis. King–Denborough syndrome describes an AD form of *RYR1*-related myopathy characterised by MH, dysmorphic features and skeletal abnormalities. Episodes of rhabdomyolysis in *RYR1*-related disease typically follow bouts of prolonged exercise in warm or hot environments and/or in situations leading to dehydration.

As previously stated, the histopathological changes in *RYR1*-related disease can be varied, ranging from the classical finding of central cores within muscle fibres ("central core disease" [CCD]) to multiminicore disease to rod-cord pathologies. Subtler forms of the disorder may simply show the isolated finding of congenital fibre-type disproportion (Figure C31.1). In some cases, typically in adults, the muscle biopsy may be normal.

The cases described here, and Case 11, exemplify the breadth of *RYR1*-related disease and emphasise the significant phenotypic and intrafamilial variability often associated with the diagnosis. Diagnosis may be further complicated by the frequent identification of variants of uncertain significance in *RYR1*. These cases may require muscle biopsy for histopathological diagnostic support.

Management of *RYR1*-related rhabdomyolysis follows standard protocols. Some experts advocate the early use of dantrolene, which is thought to lessen the severity or duration of attacks of rhabdomyolysis.

MH is a severe, potentially fatal, reaction to certain inhaled drugs used for general anaesthesia and depolarising neuromuscular blockade. The cause is an uncontrolled release of calcium from the SR leading to sustained muscle contraction and hypermetabolism. The earliest sign is increased end-tidal CO_2. MH is normally an AD inherited trait and three hotspots in *RYR1* account for most pathogenic variants. A smaller number of cases are caused by pathogenic variants in *CACNA1S* and *STAC3*. Although there are MH testing protocols (*in vitro* halothane and caffeine contracture testing on a sample of muscle) and referral centres for testing in some countries, access to such facilities is limited. Therefore, in the absence of testing facilities, a pragmatic approach is to counsel patients with

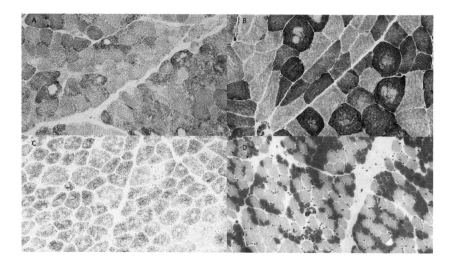

Figure C31.1 Range of findings in RYR1 myopathies. A. Succinate dehydrogenase (SDH) (10×) highlighting the presence of cores in type 1 muscle fibres. B.
Nicotinamide adenine dinucleotide (NADH) (20×) demonstrating the presence
of cores in type 1 muscle fibres. C. SDH (10×) highlighting the presence of multi-
minicores in type 1 fibres. D. Metachromatic ATPase (10×) demonstrating congenital fibre type disproportion, with the more darkly staining type 1 fibres at
least 50% smaller than the adjacent type 2 fibres. Additionally, the stain demonstrates mild myopathic grouping of fibre types.

RYR1-related disease and family members about the potential risk for MH. This
is increasingly important as cases of MH linked to pathogenic variants beyond
the three hotspots are reported and the fact that MH may occur even despite
an individual having undergone previous (and sometimes multiple) uneventful
general anaesthesia.

Learning points
- *RYR1*-related disorders comprise a phenotypically and morphologically
  diverse group of disorders.
- In the absence of access to testing facilities for MH, all patients and
  families with a pathogenic variant in *RYR1* should be counselled about
  the risk of MH.

CASE 32

Stefen Brady

History

A 71-year-old woman was referred for further management of treatment-resistant seronegative myasthenia gravis. She had presented 6 months earlier with a 4-month history of bilateral ptosis and diplopia. She was made aware of the ptosis when Her Majesty's Customs and Excise Officers repeatedly had to ask her to open her eyes while trying to use a retinal scanner to confirm her identity on her return from an overseas trip. On repeat questioning, she was adamant that her ptosis and diplopia varied throughout the day. She denied dysphagia or limb weakness and had no family history of note. Acetylcholine receptor (AChR) and muscle-specific kinase (MuSK) antibodies were not detected. Her initial neurophysiological assessment was unremarkable. Treatment with increasing doses of acetylcholinesterase inhibitor, pyridostigmine, and glucocorticoids had proved ineffective.

Examination

She was of short stature – 4'11" (143 cm) – with symmetrical ptosis and almost complete bilateral ophthalmoparesis with preservation of down-gaze. Diplopia and fatigability were not demonstrated.

Investigations

A review of her family photos revealed that she did not have ptosis 4 years earlier, but she was significantly shorter than her siblings. Her creatine kinase (CK) and serum lactate levels were mildly elevated at 377 IU/L (normal 25–200 U/L) and 2.5 mmol/l (normal 0.5–2.2 mmol/L), respectively. Electromyography (EMG) showed myopathic changes, while single-fibre studies were unremarkable. The findings from a deltoid muscle biopsy are shown in Figure C32.1.

DOI: 10.1201/9780429429323-43

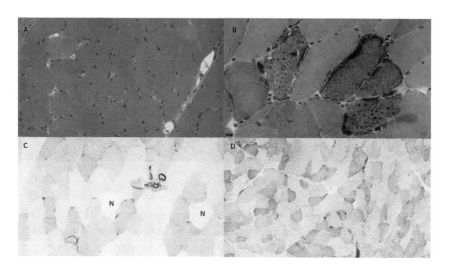

Figure C32.1 (A) Haematoxylin and eosin-stained slide demonstrating minor variation in muscle fibre diameters and the presence of a granular fibre (blue arrow) (20x). (B) Modified Gömöri trichrome showing ragged red fibres indicating peripheral accumulation of mitochondria (40x). (C) Cytochrome c oxidase (COX) histochemical stain revealing COX-negative muscle fibres (N) (20x). (D) Combined COX/succinate dehydrogenase (SDH) stain with multiple COX-negative/SDH-positive fibres (blue) (10x).

DIAGNOSIS

Chronic progressive external ophthalmoplegia (CPEO or PEO) due to a single large mitochondrial DNA deletion.

Discussion

Chronic progressive external ophthalmoplegia (CPEO/PEO) is a mitochondrial disorder typified by progressive ophthalmoparesis and ptosis. Symptoms usually develop in the fifth decade. Additional clinical features such as dysphagia, myopathy and neuropathy may also be present. Progression is slow and, as in this case, symptoms may go unnoticed by the individual and their family and friends. Two-thirds of cases of PEO are due to a single mitochondrial DNA deletion. The remainder, in descending frequency, are due to nuclear DNA pathogenic variants and mitochondrial DNA pathogenic point variants. The clinical presentation aids molecular genetic testing. For example, if a neuropathy is present in addition to PEO, the likely cause is a pathogenic variant in the nuclear DNA (1).

Primary mitochondrial diseases are caused by pathogenic variants in either mitochondrial or nuclear DNA. They are phenotypically protean. It is often said that mitochondrial diseases can present at any age and may affect any or multiple organs. The range of presenting clinical features includes diabetes mellitus, deafness, short stature, cardiomyopathy, gastrointestinal symptoms, optic neuropathy, migraine, epileptic seizures, ataxia, neuropathy and myopathy.

Mitochondrial DNA is a 16.5kb circular molecule. Multiple copies are present in each cell. It encodes 37 essential mitochondrial proteins. However, hundreds of proteins essential to mitochondrial function are encoded by nuclear DNA and transported into mitochondria. Consequently, mitochondrial diseases result from pathogenic variants in either mitochondrial or nuclear DNA, and inheritance is correspondingly maternal or autosomal. In adults, mitochondrial diseases are more frequently caused by pathogenic variants in mitochondrial DNA. The converse is true in childhood when mitochondrial diseases are more frequently due to pathogenic variants in nuclear DNA. The clinical presentation of mitochondrial disease also varies with increasing age.

Several classical mitochondrial syndromes are described, such as MERRF (myoclonic epilepsy and red ragged fibres), MELAS (mitochondrial encephalomyopathy, lactic acidosis and stroke-like episodes), NARP (neurogenic weakness, ataxia and retinitis pigmentosa) and SANDO (sensory ataxic neuropathy, dysarthria and ophthalmoplegia). Although these syndromes can aid diagnosis, individuals with mitochondrial disease often do not fit neatly into such categories. In older adults, PEO and ptosis, and myopathy are the more common presentations.

The differential diagnosis of ptosis and ophthalmoparesis in an older adult includes myasthenia gravis (MG) and oculopharyngeal muscular dystrophy (OPMD). Certain clinical features are useful in differentiating these disorders. First, true fatigable weakness is only observed in MG. Although individuals with PEO may complain of diplopia, it is not demonstrable on physical examination.

Second, inferior gaze is relatively spared in PEO. Third, individuals with PEO frequently complain of dysphagia (2). However, marked dysphagia argues against a diagnosis of PEO and is more suggestive of MG and OPMD.

Management of mitochondrial disease is largely supportive with no curative treatment available. It includes surveillance for weight loss and dysphagia, hearing loss, cardiac disease (rhythm disturbances and cardiomyopathy), endocrine dysfunction such as diabetes mellitus, and ophthalmological abnormalities including ptosis and retinopathy. Despite the absence of an effective treatment, identification of the genetic cause is hugely important to individuals and families affected by mitochondrial diseases, as it enables accurate genetic counselling and guidance on reproductive options.

Learning points

- Mitochondrial diseases are common (affecting 1 in 4300 adults) (3), and clinically (phenotypically) and genetically heterogeneous.
- Multisystem involvement is the rule but is not invariable.
- Classic clinical syndromes such as MELAS and MERRF aid diagnosis and can help guide molecular genetic testing.
- The main differential diagnoses of PEO in an older adult are MG or OPMD. Subacute onset, fatigable weakness on examination, early and marked paresis of inferior gaze and severe bulbar involvement argue against a diagnosis of mitochondrial disease.
- Management is largely supportive and involves surveillance for complications of mitochondrial disease such as cataracts, deafness, diabetes mellitus and cardiac disease.

Further reading

1. Horga A, *et al.* Peripheral neuropathy predicts nuclear gene defect in patients with mitochondrial ophthalmoplegia. *Brain.* 2014;137:3200–12.
2. Hedermann G, Løkken N, Dahlqvist JR, Vissing J. Dysphagia is prevalent in patients with CPEO and single, large-scale deletions in mtDNA. *Mitochondrion.* 2017;32:27–30.
3. Gorman GS, Schaefer AM, Ng Y, Gomez N, Blakely EL, Alston CL, et al. Prevalence of nuclear and mitochondrial DNA mutations related to adult mitochondrial disease. *Ann Neurol.* 2015;77(5):753–9.

Case 33

Stefen Brady

History

A 53-year-old man was acutely admitted to hospital via accident and emergency, several months prior to his presentation to clinic, with a possible stroke. His partner described that his symptoms started several days earlier with a severe generalised headache and vomiting. He had a history of classical migraine without aura. Over the following days prior to admission, he developed an expressive dysphasia and appeared increasingly confused. He was admitted to the stroke ward, where he received standard treatment for an ischaemic stroke. He recovered over a period of several weeks and was discharged home.

Further enquiry revealed that he had lost his hearing in his 30s and had a family history of maternal deafness. There was no other personal or family history of note.

Examination

He was cachectic with asymmetric ptosis (right greater than left), incongruous right homonymous hemianopia, marked ophthalmoparesis in all directions and unaccompanied by diplopia. He had difficulty rising from a seated position due to mild weakness of hip flexion, and cerebellar ataxia affecting the upper and lower limbs.

Investigations

Investigations, including full blood count, renal profile, HbA1c, lipid profile and creatine kinase (CK), were normal except for a raised serum lactate of 6.5 mmol/L.

A review of his stroke imaging identified T2 high signal in the left temporal lobe with extension into the insular cortex and restricted diffusion with diffusion-weighted imaging (DWI). Repeat imaging several weeks later showed progression of the T2 high signal to involve the right frontal and left occipital lobes.

DOI: 10.1201/9780429429323-44

DIAGNOSIS

Mitochondrial encephalomyopathy, lactic acidosis and stroke-like episodes (MELAS). Genetic testing for the m.3243A>G point mutation showed that the individual had 19% heteroplasmy in blood and 88% in urine.

Discussion

The dual genetic control of mitochondria means that primary mitochondrial disease is the result of pathogenic variants in either nuclear or mitochondrial DNA (mtDNA). As a result, the pattern of inheritance associated with mitochondrial diseases is autosomal (dominant or recessive) or maternal. Although considered to be rare, prevalence studies have shown that 1 in 400–500 individuals in the population carry the pathogenic mtDNA point variant, m.3243A>G (1), which is also the commonest cause of MELAS, and 1 in 100 individuals harbour a single pathogenic variant in the mitochondrial polymerase *POLG* (2–4). However, most individuals carrying the pathogenic mtDNA point variant m.3243A>G are asymptomatic because the level of mitochondrial heteroplasmy (the ratio of normal "wild-type" mitochondrial DNA to pathogenic mitochondrial DNA) is below disease-causing threshold. This threshold varies for different mitochondrial point variants (5–7).

MELAS is the prototypical mitochondrial disease. It is multisystem, of variable severity and maternally inherited. As described earlier, the disease severity is related to the degree of heteroplasmy, which varies between tissues. The level of heteroplasmy in blood declines with increasing age. Thus, in adults, the level is quantified from urinary epithelial cells or skeletal muscle. The canonical clinical features associated with MELAS are progressive external ophthalmoparesis (PEO), hearing loss, epilepsy, ataxia, diabetes mellitus, cardiomyopathy, and stroke-like episodes (SLEs). In general, management of the medical and neurological complications of MELAS is little different from their management in the absence of mitochondrial disease.

The most severe and dramatic clinical feature of MELAS is the SLE. Although relatively quick in evolution, SLEs, unlike a true ischaemic stroke, progress over several days and initial symptoms often include headache, nausea and vomiting, confusion (encephalopathy), and seizures. MRI of the brain often shows T2 high signal in the occipital lobes and extending across vascular territories. The pathogenesis of a SLE is not ischaemic but metabolic failure. Whether clinically apparent or not, a SLE is typically driven by ongoing seizure activity. Therefore, urgent electroencephalography (EEG) and aggressive management of seizure activity are of primary importance, along with treatment of any concomitant infection and ensuring appropriate hydration and adequate calorie intake. Pharmacological management of seizures associated with MELAS should follow local protocols, except sodium valproate is best avoided when the genotype is unknown. Gastrointestinal pseudo-obstruction can complicate SLEs and should be actively sought. Currently, there is no convincing evidence to support the use of mitochondrial-specific treatments such as ubiquinone (coenzyme Q10), ribo-flavin or L-arginine.

MELAS and the mitochondrial pathogenic point mutation m.3243A>G are, like many clinical syndromes and genes, associated with genotypic and pheno-typic variability, respectively. M.3243A>G is the single most frequent cause of MELAS, accounting for 80% of cases. The remaining 20% of cases are associ-ated with other pathogenic mitochondrial DNA point variants and the nuclear gene encoding the sole mitochondrial DNA polymerase, *POLG*. Phenotypes associated with m.3243A>G, in addition to MELAS, are PEO, Leigh syndrome, maternally inherited diabetes and deafness (MIDD), and isolated myopathy. Phenotypic variation can be observed in a family with m.3243A>G and relates to an individual's level of heteroplasmy.

Diagnosing mitochondrial disease is complicated by its clinical heterogeneity, variable inheritance and, despite earlier comment, relative rarity. Having sus-pected mitochondrial disease, investigation is not without complexity. First, although certain test results may support a diagnosis of mitochondrial disease such as a raised serum lactate, mitochondrial abnormalities on muscle biopsy (ragged red muscle fibres or cytochrome c oxidase [COX] negative/succinate dehydrogenase [SDH] positive muscle fibres), basal ganglia calcification on head CT, or white matter changes on MRI, they lack sensitivity and specificity. Bar genetic analysis, there is no gold-standard test for mitochondrial disease. Second, genetic testing for mitochondrial disease involves selection of the correct tissue sample (blood, urine or muscle) for testing and the most appropriate initial test, which may be testing for a common pathogenic point variant in mtDNA, mito-chondrial DNA depletion or deletions, or assessment for nuclear DNA causes of mitochondrial disease. High throughput genetic sequencing has dramatically changed the pathway for investigating mitochondrial disease and the need for invasive tests such as muscle biopsy, so it is recommended to discuss the appro-priate testing for suspected mitochondrial disease with a mitochondrial disease specialist and local mitochondrial genetic laboratory.

Learning points

- Mitochondrial disease should be considered in a multisystem disor-der, particularly if ptosis and ophthalmoparesis, hearing loss, epilepsy, ataxia, or peripheral neuropathy are present.
- Inheritance of mitochondrial disease is varied and identification of the clinical syndrome, such as MELAS, helps to direct genetic testing.
- Clinical features supportive of a SLE are subacute onset and neurologi-cal progression, headache, nausea and vomiting, confusion, and positive neurological symptoms.
- SLEs are seizure-driven and require aggressive anticonvulsant treatment.

Further reading

1. Manwaring N, Jones MM, Wang JJ, Rochtchina E, Howard C, Mitchell P, et al. Population prevalence of the MELAS A3243G mutation. *Mitochondrion.* 2007;7(3):230–3.
2. Winterthun S, Ferrari G, He L, Taylor RW, Zeviani M, Turnbull DM, et al. Autosomal recessive mitochondrial ataxic syndrome due to mitochondrial polymerase gamma mutations. *Neurology.* 2005;64(7):1204–8.
3. Hakonen AH, Heiskanen S, Juvonen V, Lappalainen I, Luoma PT, Rantamäki M, et al. Mitochondrial DNA polymerase W748S mutation: A common cause of autosomal recessive ataxia with ancient European origin. *Am J Hum Genet.* 2005;77(3):430–41.
4. Horvath R, Hudson G, Ferrari G, Fütterer N, Ahola S, Lamantea E, et al. Phenotypic spectrum associated with mutations of the mitochondrial polymerase gamma gene. *Brain J Neurol.* 2006;129(Pt 7):1674–84.
5. Ng YS, Martikainen MH, Gorman GS, Blain A, Bugiardini E, Bunting A, et al. Pathogenic variants in MT-ATP6: A United Kingdom–based mitochondrial disease cohort study. *Ann Neurol.* 2019;86(2):310–5.
6. Nesbitt V, Pitceathly RDS, Turnbull DM, Taylor RW, Sweeney MG, Mudanohwo EE, et al. The UK MRC Mitochondrial Disease Patient Cohort Study: clinical phenotypes associated with the m.3243A>G mutation—implications for diagnosis and management. *J Neurol Neurosurg Psychiatry.* 2013;84(8):936–8.
7. Gorman GS, Schaefer AM, Ng Y, Gomez N, Blakely EL, Alston CL, et al. Prevalence of nuclear and mitochondrial DNA mutations related to adult mitochondrial disease. *Ann Neurol.* 2015;77(5):753–9.
8. Mavraki E, Labrum R, Sergeant K. et al. Genetic testing for mitochondrial disease: the United Kingdom best practice guidelines. *Eur J Hum Genet* 2023;31:148–63.
9. Ng YS, Bindoff LA, Gorman GS, Horvath R, Klopstock T, Mancuso M, Martikainen MH, Mcfarland R, Nesbitt V, Pitceathly RDS, Schaefer AM, Turnbull DM. Consensus-based statements for the management of mitochondrial stroke-like episodes. *Wellcome Open Res.* 2019 Dec 13;4:201.

CASE 34

Stefen Brady

History

A 58-year-old man was seen in the neuromuscular clinic after reporting symptoms of increasing lower limb weakness which had developed over a period of 12 to 18 months. In adolescence, after presenting with lower limb weakness, he had been given a diagnosis of tubular aggregate myopathy (TAM) following a muscle biopsy. He was subsequently lost to follow-up for over 30 years.

At his current presentation, he denied the presence of ocular, orobulbar or cardio-respiratory symptoms, nor did he report any fatigable symptoms. He described himself as physically unlike the rest of his family. While most of his family were stocky and athletic, he was slim and had never been good at sports. He had no other family history of note.

Examination

Cranial nerve examination was normal. He had slim limb muscles with moderate weakness of shoulder abduction and hip flexion (MRC grading 3/5) as well as mild weakness of elbow extension and flexion, finger extension, knee extension and ankle dorsiflexion (4/5). There was no fatigable weakness of the ocular, orobulbar or limb muscles.

Investigations

The creatine kinase (CK) was normal (96 U/L, normal 40–320 IU/L). Electromyography (EMG) showed small, short-duration polyphasic units. Repetitive nerve stimulation (RNS) of the right median, ulnar and spinal accessory nerves showed decrement of the compound action muscle potential greater than 10% and single fibre electromyography (SFEMG) revealed jitter and blocking. A muscle biopsy (Figure C34.1) performed when the patient was 15 years old showed frequent large sarcoplasmic tubular aggregates in type I and II fibres on light microscopy, the presence of which was confirmed with electron microscopy (EM) (Figure C34.2).

Follow-up

The patient was commenced on the acetylcholinesterase inhibitor pyridostigmine. This led to an improvement in his limb weakness. Later 3,4-diamino-pyridine (3,4-DAP) was added to his medication regimen with additional symptomatic benefit.

DOI: 10.1201/9780429429323-45

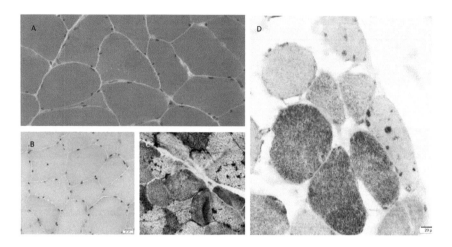

Figure C34.1 (A) Haematoxylin and eosin stain showing mild muscle fibre size variation and atrophy with occasional fibres showing irregular internal slits and vacuoles. These appear clear in this case but may contain eosinophilic material in other cases (40x). (B) Modified Gömöri trichrome highlighting the small slits and vacuoles within the muscle fibres, which do, in such cases, often contain red material (40x). (C) With nicotinamide adenine dinucleotide (NADH) histochemical staining, the material within the slits and vacuoles is strongly positive (40x). (D) sarco-/endoplasmic reticulum Ca^{2+}-ATPase (SERCA1) immunohistochemical staining shows positive staining within the slits and vacuoles (40x).

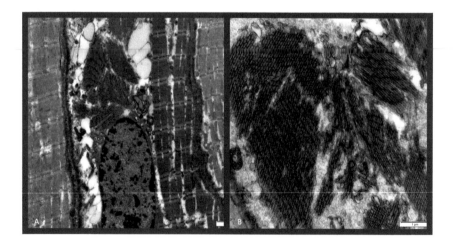

Figure C34.2 (A) Electron microscopy (EM) demonstrating the presence of 70 to 400 nm tubules with central dense material in muscle fibres. (B) EM at 1 μm highlighting the structure of tubules. A number of different forms of TAs are described.

DIAGNOSIS

Limb girdle congenital myasthenic syndrome (LG-CMS) due to compound heterozygous mutations in *DPAGT1*.

Discussion

The combination of limb girdle weakness, neurophysiological evidence of impairment of the neuromuscular junction and the presence of tubular aggregates (TAs) on muscle biopsy is consistent with a diagnosis of LG-CMS.

Congenital myasthenic syndromes (CMS) are a group of rare, mostly autosomal recessive disorders characterised by fatigable weakness and neurophysiological evidence of abnormality of the neuromuscular junction. At this time, more than 20 genes have been identified in association with CMS. In the UK, 70% of cases are due to acetylcholine receptor (AChR) deficiency and pathogenic variants in *DOK7* and *RAPSYN* (1).

LG-CMS is a discreet group of CMS with prominent limb girdle weakness and minimal or no craniobulbar involvement. Consequently, LG-CMS may be misdiagnosed as a muscular dystrophy. Adult-onset LG-CMS is associated with pathogenic variants in genes encoding proteins involved in glycosylation, most frequently *GFPT1* and *DPAGT1* and rarely *ALG2*, *ALG14* and *GMPPB*.

CK can be normal or markedly raised in patients with LG-CMS, the latter further attributing to misdiagnosis. Neurophysiological evidence of neuromuscular junction dysfunction should be sought in the proximal muscles in LG-CMS, otherwise it may be missed. TAs on muscle biopsy are well described in LG-CMS due to mutations in *GFPT1*, *DPAGT1* and *ALG2*. Additional reported pathological features include the presence of vacuoles and reduced α-dystroglycan staining of muscle sarcolemma.

Treatments for LG-CMS include acetylcholinesterase inhibitors such as pyridostigmine; 3,4-DAP, which blocks presynaptic potassium channels increasing the amount of acetylcholine within the neuromuscular junction; and β-adrenoceptor agonist salbutamol, which is clinically efficacious, however, its mechanism of action at the neuromuscular junction is uncertain.

As previously stated, CMS and LG-CMS may be misdiagnosed as muscular dystrophy, particularly when symptoms and signs of fatigability are limited or subtle, and investigations such as CK levels, neurophysiology and muscle biopsy may be misleading. However, in any patient with clinical or neurophysiological evidence of muscle fatigability, it is important to first consider a diagnosis of autoimmune myasthenia gravis (MG) prior to CMS, as the prevalence of MG is roughly 10–40 times greater than CMS. Clinical features that favour a diagnosis of CMS rather than MG are the childhood onset of symptoms and distal weakness.

Learning points

- LG-CMS is a discreet group of CMS that can be confused with muscular dystrophy because of minimal craniobulbar signs and fatigability with marked limb girdle weakness.
- Adult-onset LG-CMS is associated with pathogenic variants in genes involved in the glycosylation pathway.
- Autoimmune MG is much more common than CMS and should always be considered first in patients with clinical or neurophysiological evidence of fatigable weakness.

Further reading

1. Rodríguez Cruz PM, Palace J, Beeson D. The neuromuscular junction and wide heterogeneity of congenital myasthenic syndromes. *Int J Mol Sci.* 2018; 19:1677.

Case 35

Andria Merrison

PATIENT ASSESSMENT

History

A 22-year-old man presented with progressive difficulty with walking and standing from a seated position. He had also noticed thinning of the muscles in his legs over several years. He did not report any sensory or other neurological symptoms.

Whilst he had reached normal motor milestones in early childhood and attended physical education lessons at school, he had never enjoyed sport. He had been described as a clumsy child. He had no other significant medical history.

Examination

All cranial nerves were intact. There was symmetrical thinning of the quadriceps and hamstrings bilaterally. There were a few fasciculations seen in proximal muscles in all four limbs. Tone, reflexes and co-ordination were normal and plantars flexor Sensory function was normal.

Investigations

Creatine kinase (CK) was 542 U/L. Nerve conduction studies showed normal sensory nerve action potentials and low amplitude compound muscle action potentials. Electromyography showed features of denervation (fibrillation potentials, positive sharp waves and fasciculation potentials) as well as re-innervation (decreased numbers of motor unit potentials with increased amplitude and prolonged duration).

Genetic testing identified a deletion in the SMN1 gene. SMN copy number was 3.

DOI: 10.1201/9780429429323-46

DIAGNOSIS

Spinal muscular atrophy.

Discussion

Spinal muscular atrophy (SMA) is an autosomal recessive condition characterised by degeneration of motor nerves. It is the commonest disorder of motor nerves in childhood, with an incidence of 1/10,000 live births. In adults, amyotrophic lateral sclerosis (ALS) is the most common condition to affect motor nerves. SMA is discussed here as the distinction between muscle conditions, SMA and ALS can be difficult, and SMA is an important differential in patients with neuromuscular problems.

SMA is caused by deletion, gene conversion or occasionally point mutation of the survival motor neurone gene (SMN1). This leads to a severe reduction in SMN protein levels, which in turn leads to degeneration of lower motor neurones (although the details of the mechanism for degeneration are unclear). SMN plays a critical role in the assembly of small nuclear ribonucleoproteins (snRNPs), which are essential for pre-mRNA splicing.

The SMN2 gene, which is an almost identical paralogue of SMN1 that has arisen due to evolutionary duplication, produces small amounts of residual protein, which is protective and prevents the lethal outcome of complete loss of SMN protein. Disease severity is proportional to the remaining SMN levels, which is largely determined by SMN2 copy number.

Three main forms of SMA are recognised based on clinical presentation:

	Age of onset	Number of SMN2 copies	Clinical features
SMA type I	Infantile	2	Floppy infant Never able to sit Without gene therapy, death at <2 years
SMA type II	>6 months	3	Able to sit (but may lose this ability) Never able to walk unaided Kyphoscoliosis usually occurs Bulbar involvement common Respiratory muscle weakness develops in all
SMA type III	<3 years, SMA type IIIa >3 years, SMA type IIIb	3, SMA type IIIa 4, SMA type IIIb	Able to walk unaided but lose ambulation Most patients with SMA IIIa lose ambulation by 14 years, without gene therapy Kyphoscoliosis can occur

In very severe cases, onset is in utero (type 0) and fetal hypotonia can lead to arthrogryposis. There is also a milder form of the disease (type IV) with onset in adulthood, which is slowly progressive. Those with adult-onset SMA are a genetically heterogeneous group and can present with varying degrees of severity early in adult life.

Gene-modifying therapy is now available for people living with SMA. Currently, the two licensed therapies are nusinersen (which is delivered by regular intrathecal injections – a loading regimen, followed by three injections per year) and risdiplam (an oral agent supplied as a liquid and taken daily). These treatments have had excellent early outcomes (with regard to improved muscle strength in the limbs, trunk and respiratory muscle function) for babies and children presenting with SMA. Their efficacy long term and for patients presenting in adult life is being assessed. Further gene replacement therapy trials are underway, including onasemnogene abeparvovec.

A number of countries now provide routine newborn screening for SMA. In view of the benefits of early intervention with gene therapy, there is a case for these programmes to be delivered worldwide.

In making the distinction between SMA and ALS in adults, patients with SMA tend to be younger at the onset of symptoms, have early symmetrical involvement of muscles, have frequent early restriction to specific anatomical territories (e.g. lower limbs) and show slower progression over years or decades. Those who survive into adulthood have later onset bulbar and respiratory problems but most do go on to develop these complications over time.

Learning points
- Spinal muscular atrophy is an autosomal recessive condition, due to mutations in the SMN1 gene, which is the commonest disorder of motor nerves in childhood but can present in early adult life.
- It is an important differential diagnosis to consider in patients presenting with muscle wasting. Signs of denervation, including fasciculation, may be evident.
- Without gene therapy, patients with the infantile form die before the age of 2 years and those with childhood onset usually lose ambulation by 14 years.
- Gene-modifying therapy is now available for people living with SMA: nusinersen (intrathecal injection) and risdiplam (oral medication).

Further reading
Aragon-Gawinska K, Mouraux C, Dangouloff T, Servais L. 2023. Spinal muscular atrophy treatment in patients identified by newborn screening – a systematic review. *Genes* 29; 14(7): 1377.

Mercuri E, Finkel RS, Muntoni F, Wirth B, Montes, J, Main M, Mazzone ES, Vitale M, Snyder B, Quijano-Roy S, Bertini E, Hurst Davis R, Meyer OH, Simonds AK, Schroth MK, Graham RJ, Kirschner J, Iannaccone ST, Crawford TO,

Woods S, Qian Y, Sejersen T. 2018. Diagnosis and management of spinal muscular atrophy: Part 1: Recommendations for diagnosis, rehabilitation, orthopaedic and nutritional care. *Neuromuscular Disorders* 28(2): 103–115.

Mercuri E, Finkel RS, Muntoni F, Wirth B, Montes, J, Main M, Mazzone ES, Vitale M, Snyder B, Quijano-Roy S, Bertini E, Hurst Davis R, Meyer OH, Simonds AK, Schroth MK, Graham RJ, Kirschner J, Iannaccone ST, Crawford TO, Woods S, Qian Y, Sejersen T. 2018. Diagnosis and management of spinal muscular atrophy: Part 2: Pulmonary and acute care; medications, supplements and immunizations; other organ systems and ethics. *Neuromuscular Disorders* 28(3): 197–207.

Mercuri E, Sumner CJ, Muntoni F, Darras BT & Finkel RS. 2022. Spinal muscular atrophy. *Nature Reviews Disease Primers* 8(1): 52.

Nishio H, Niba ETE, Saito T, Okamoto K, Takeshima Y & Awano H. 2023. Spinal muscular atrophy: the past, present and future of diagnosis and treatment. *International Journal of Molecular Sciences* 24(15): 11939.

Schorling DC, Pechmann A, Kirschner J. 2020 Advances in treatment of spinal muscular atrophy – new phenotypes, new challenges, new implications for care. *Journal of Neuromuscular Disorders* 7: 1–13.

CASE 36

Andria Merrison

History

A 36-year-old man presented with a 5-year history of reduced exercise tolerance with his ankles giving way at times. He had increasing cramps, particularly in the calf muscles. Walking upstairs was difficult and he had recently had a few falls. He had also experienced some mild weakness and occasional pins and needles in the hands. He had noticed thinning of the muscles in the hands, feet and calves. He reported mild problems with chewing and occasional difficulties with swallowing.

There was no significant past medical history or family history.

Examination

There was mild neck flexion weakness but no other cranial nerve abnormality. He had a fine tremor in both hands. Tone was normal. There was mild weakness in all muscle groups, worse distally than proximally. Distal symmetrical wasting in all four limbs was evident. Ankle jerks were absent but other reflexes were preserved and plantars were downgoing. Sensory function was intact.

With time, this man's symptoms worsened and he developed problems with chewing and occasional swallowing difficulties. His sleep pattern was very poor, repeatedly waking in the night and feeling fatigued during the day. Fasciculations became evident in the face, trunk and all four limbs.

Investigations

Creatine kinase (CK) was raised at 1600 U/L and alanine aminotransferase (ALT) at 68 U/L. All other blood tests were normal. Neurophysiological testing showed mixed neurogenic and myopathic changes, nerve conduction studies showed low sensory nerve amplitudes and decreased compound motor action potentials, and electromyography showed evidence of denervation. A muscle biopsy was performed. This revealed a combination of muscle fibre necrosis and regeneration with associated interstitial fibrosis; changes initially thought to be due to a muscular dystrophy (Figure C36.1). Immunohistochemistry for both muscular dystrophies and myofibrillar myopathies was negative.

Lung function tests and overnight oximetry revealed respiratory muscle weakness and nocturnal hypoventilation. Repeat neurophysiological investigations were consistent with anterior horn cell dysfunction. Genetic testing confirmed the diagnosis.

DOI: 10.1201/9780429429323-47

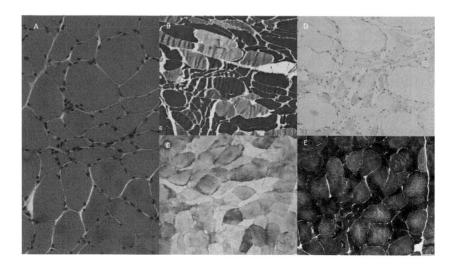

Figure C36.1 Chronic Partial Denervation. A. H&E 10× demonstrating areas of group fibre atrophy composed of angulated atrophic fibres. B. Metachromatic ATPase 10× highlighting group fibre atrophy of type 1 fibres without fibre type grouping. C. PAS 10× showing loss of glycogen content in denervated angulated fibres (a soft sign of denervation). D. nNOS 10× immunostaining demonstrating loss of sarcolemmal expression in denervated fibres. E. NADH 10× highlighting an increase in staining concentration in Type 1 (dark) angulated atrophic/denervated fibres.

DIAGNOSIS

Kennedy's disease.

Discussion

Spinal and bulbar muscular atrophy, also known as Kennedy's disease, is an adult-onset neurodegenerative condition affecting motor neurones in the brain-stem and spinal cord (Kennedy 1968). It is caused by a trinucleotide (CAG) repeat expansion in the androgen receptor (AR) gene on the X chromosome (La Spada 1991); longer repeats cause earlier onset but not more rapid progression. There is an androgen-dependent toxic gain of function in the resultant mutant protein which affects transcription and other cellular mechanisms in both motor neurones and muscles. Prevalence is about 1 in 40,000. Most patients present in the third or fourth decade of life.

Weakness occurs in both proximal and distal muscles of the upper and lower limbs. The presentation may be asymmetric (Rhodes 2009). Dysarthria (nasal speech), dysphagia and facial weakness may be present. There may be lower motor neurone signs, including decreased or absent tendon reflexes and fascicu-lations (including in the face and tongue) (Breza 2018). Some patients have sen-sory symptoms as a consequence of dorsal root ganglion degeneration. Androgen insensitivity may manifest as gynaecomastia, reduced fertility and erectile dys-function. This condition is easily misdiagnosed as amyotrophic lateral sclerosis (ALS), but the absence of upper motor neurone signs and the additional features of Kennedy's disease may provide clues (Manzono 2018).

Genetic testing is diagnostic. Ninety per cent of patients have a raised CK (900–1400 IU/L). Nerve conduction studies usually demonstrate decreased compound motor action potentials and reduced sensory amplitudes. Electromyography usu-ally shows evidence of denervation. Muscle biopsy is not necessary to establish a diagnosis but typically shows features of chronic partial denervation, with group fibre atrophy without fibre type grouping (Figure C36.1B). Increased internal nuclei and pyknotic nuclear clusters may also be seen. However, genetic testing is diagnostic for Kennedy's disease.

Aspartate aminotransferase (AST) and LDL levels may be raised, and impaired glucose tolerance can be associated with this condition. The hormone profile may be altered: raised total testosterone; free testosterone, dihydrotestosterone and oestradiol; and reduced androstenedione (Rosenbohm 2018). (Although a minority may have reduced androgen levels.)

Two-thirds of patients have a positive family history. Being X-linked, it is a disor-der in males but a minority of females present as partially manifesting carriers, usually presenting with muscle cramps (Isihara 2001). Genetic counselling, pre-implantation and prenatal genetic testing are available.

Progression is typically slow (losing around 2% of muscle strength per year), a third of patients require a wheelchair 20 years after diagnosis and many patients have a normal life span. Patients with higher testosterone levels may have better muscle strength and quality of life. There is currently no curative treatment and management focuses on preventing/treating the complications of the disease (including respiratory support) and maintaining function through exercise, physiotherapy and good nutrition.

Learning points

- Consider Kennedy's disease in a male patient with slowly progressive wasting and fasciculations without upper motor neurone signs.
- Gynaecomastia is present in a number of cases.
- A minority of females present as partially manifesting carriers, with muscle cramps.

Further reading

Breza M & Koutis G. (2018) Spinal and bulbar muscular atrophy (Kennedy disease): a clinically orientated review of a rare disease. *Journal of Neurology* 266(3): 565–573.

Grunseich C, Fischbeck KH. (2020) Molecular pathogenesis of spinal muscular atrophy (Kennedy's disease) and avenues for treatment. *Current Opinion Neurology* 33(5): 629–34.

Isihara H, Kanda F, Nishio H et al. (2001) Clinical features and skewed X-chromosome inactivation in female carriers of X-linked recessive spinal and bulbar muscular atrophy. *Journal of Neurology* 248: 856–60.

Kennedy WR, Alter M & Sung JH. (1968) Progressive proximal spinal and bulbar muscular atrophy of late onset: a sex-linked recessive trait. *Neurology* 18: 671–80.

La Spada AR, Wilson EM, Lubahn DB, Harding AE & Fischbeck KH. (1991) Androgen receptor gene mutations in X-linked spinal and bulbar muscular atrophy. *Nature* 352: 77–9.

Manzono R, Soraru G, Grunseich C, Fratta P, Zuccaro E, Pennuto M & Rinaldi C. (2018) Beyond motor neurones: expanding the clinical spectrum in Kennedy's disease. *Journal of Neurology, Neurosurgery and Neuropsychiatry* 89(8): 808–12.

Marchioretti C, Andreotti R, Zuccaro E, Lieberman AP, Basso M, Pennuto M. (2023) Spinal and bulbar muscular atrophy: From molecular pathogenesis to pharmacological intervention targeting skeletal muscle. *Current Opinion Pharmacology* 71: 102394.

Rhodes LE, Freeman BK, Auh S et al. (2009) Clinical features of spinal and bulbar muscular atrophy. *Brain* 132: 3242–51.

Rosenbohm A, Hirsch S, Volk AE, Grehl T, Grosskreutz J, Hanisch F, Herrmann A, Kollewe K, Kress W, Meyer T, Petri S, Prudlo J, Wessig C, Muller HP, Dreyhaupt J, Weishaupt J, Kubisch C, Kassubek J, Weydt P & Ludolph AC. (2018) The metabolic and endocrine characteristics in spinal and bulbar muscular atrophy. *Journal of Neurology* 265(5): 1026–1036.

INDEX

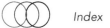